Heart Sounds and Murmurs

Heart Sounds

and

Murmurs

A Practical Guide

Second Edition

Barbara Erickson, Ph.D., R.N., CCRN
Research Analyst and Educator,
Department of Medicine Research and Education, Inc.,
Youngstown, Ohio

with 59 illustrations

 Mosby
Year Book

St. Louis   Baltimore   Boston   Chicago   London   Philadelphia   Sydney   Toronto

Mosby
Year Book

Dedicated to Publishing Excellence

Executive Editor: Don Ladig
Managing Editor: Robin Carter
Project Manager: Lin A. Dempsey
Manuscript Editor: Mary E. Drone
Production: Joan M. Herron
Book and Cover Design: Jeanne Wolfgeher
Cover Illustrator: David J. Mascaro and Associates

Library of Congress Cataloging in Publication Data

Erickson, Barbara
    Heart sounds and murmurs.

    Bibliography: p.
    Includes index.
    1. Heart—Sounds. 2. Heart—Diseases—Diagnosis.
3. Heart Murmurs—Diagnosis. I. Title. [DNLM: 1. Heart
Auscultation—programmed instruction. WG 18 E68h]
RC683.5.A9E73   1991   616.1´2   87-28238
ISBN 0-8016-6466-7

PL 9 8 7 6 5 4 3 2 1

To

Leonard P. Caccamo, M.D., F.A.C.P., F.A.C.C.

Mentor, Friend, and Inspiration

and

Frank C. Tiberio, M.D.

Clinician and Auscultator Extraordinare

Preface

The Second edition of this book is written to provide expanded information and interpretations over that found in the first edition. The basic intent and format of the book remains unchanged.

Cardiac auscultation is coming into prominence again and being recognized as an important diagnostic tool along side more modern technologies such as scans, echos or dopplers. The information derived from a properly used stethoscope is invaluable. In the hands of an individual prepared to use it, the stethoscope is a cost-effective, cost-containing invaluable instrument.

Proficiency in cardiac auscultation does not come with the acquisition of an expensive stethoscope. The most important prerequisite for effective auscultation is a prepared mind. The clinician should be aware of the dynamics of the cardiac cycle during auscultation and integrate each heart sound and murmur heard with a corresponding hemodynamic effect. This book will provide basic information on listening to and interpreting heart sounds.

Barbara Erickson

Preface to First Edition

This program is intended for the beginning auscultator who wishes to learn the basics of listening to and interpreting heart sounds. The more advanced auscultator may find the program helpful as a review of the basics.

The format used is one which has proven successful to the author over many years of teaching heart sounds. Basic information in the text is accompanied by an audio tape. By first reading the text and then listening to the tape, the learner should have the essential information necessary to understand and recognize the normal heart sounds and the most common abnormal sounds.

This book is intended as an introduction and a guide to learning heart sounds. To become clinically proficient in heart sound recognition, the learner must continually listen to as many hearts as possible. However good the reproduction of heart sounds on the tape may be, the tape can never replace the experience of listening to actual heart sounds. Please remember that the sounds on the tape have been distinctly simulated to facilitate learning. Sounds from real hearts will be similar but never heard as clearly as those on the tape.

The tape was made with a heart sound simulator using studio recording equipment.

Instructions For Use

The learner is advised to:

1. Read the basic information found in the text regarding the sound.
2. Listen to the sound on the accompanying audio tape. The tape should be repeatedly listened to until the learner is able to discern the sound being described. Before proceeding to the next section the learner must understand and *identify* each sound being described.
3. Listen to the tape with a stethoscope placed about 4 inches from the speaker. For best results, the tape should be played on a quality tape recorder. The better the sound transmission of the recorder, the better the learner will be able to hear subtle differences on the heart sound tape.
4. Listen to real hearts. Practice and repeat practice listening to heart sounds in order to gain proficiency and expertise.
5. Test their own knowledge of the content of each chapter by:
   a. Comparing behavioral objectives given at the beginning of each chapter with their own abilities on completing the chapter.
   b. Answering self-learning questions at the end of each chapter Checking their answers against those in the answer key.
   c. Listening to the "unknowns" on the tape at the end of each chapter. Checking their answers against those in the answer key.
6. Refer to the audio tape when the symbol ❖ appears in the margin.

Contents

Chapter 1

Introduction   1

    Learning Objectives   1

    History   2

    Requirements for Auscultation   2

    Cardiac Cycle   7

    Cardiac Sound-Cycle Relationship   8

    Cardiac Valve Areas   8

    Cardiac Sound Production   8

    Characteristics of Sound   9

    Sound Transmission   10

    Classification of Sounds and Murmurs   12

    Charting Heart Sounds   13

    Mimicking Sounds   15

    Self-Learning Questions   16

    Answers to Self-Learning Questions   17

Chapter 2

The First Heart Sound (S_1) 19

    Learning Objectives   19

    Components of S_1 20

    Split S_1 20

    Intensity of First Sound (S_1)   21

    Differentiating of S_1 From S_2 24

    Clinical Correlation   25

    Self-Learning "Unknown" Heart Sounds   26

    Self-Learning Questions   26

Answers to Self-Learning "Unknown" Heart Sounds   27

Answers to Self-Learning Questions   27

Chapter 3

The Second Heart Sound (S_2)   29

Learning Objectives   29

Components of S_2 30

Physiological Split S_2 30

S_2 Auscultatory Variations   31

Intensity of S_2 31

Normal S_1 and S_2 32

Clinical Correlation   32

Self-Learning "Unknown" Heart Sounds   33

Self-Learning Questions   33

Answers to Self-Learning "Unknown" Heart Sounds   34

Answers to Self-Learning Questions   34

Chapter 4

Fourth Heart Sound (S_4)   35

Learning Objectives   35

Nomenclature of S_4 36

Components of S_4 36

Differentiating S_4 From Split S_1 37

Clinical Correlation   38

Self-Learning "Unknown" Heart Sounds   38

Self-Learning Questions   39

Answers to Self-Learning "Unknown" Heart Sounds   40

Answers to Self-Learning Questions   40

Chapter 5

The Third Heart Sound (S$_3$)   *41*

Learning Objectives   41

Nomenclature of S$_3$ 42

Components of S$_3$ 42

Differentiating S$_3$ From S$_4$ 42

Clinical Correlation   43

Self-Learning "Unknown" Heart Sounds   43

Self-Learning Questions   44

Answers to Self-Learning "Unknown" Heart Sounds   45

Answers to Self-Learning Questions   45

Chapter 6

Murmurs—General Information   47

Learning Objectives   47

Characteristics of Murmurs   48

Location of Murmurs   48

Loudness of Murmurs   48

Frequency of Murmurs   49

Quality of Murmurs   50

Timing of Murmurs   50

Radiation of Murmurs   51

Shape of Murmurs   51

Special Maneuvers   52

Self-Learning "Unknown" Heart Sounds   53

Self-Learning Questions   53

Answers to Self-Learning "Unknown" Heart Sounds   54

Answers to Self-Learning Questions   54

Chapter 7

Systolic Murmurs   55

Learning Objectives   55

Mechanism of Systolic Murmur Production   56

Early Systolic Murmurs   56

Midsystolic Murmurs   57

Late Systolic Murmurs   57

Pansystolic (or Holosystolic) Murmur   57

Clinical Correlation   58

Self-Learning "Unknown" Heart Sounds   59

Self-Learning Questions   59

Answers to Self-Learning "Unknown" Heart Sounds   61

Answers to Self-Learning Questions   61

Chapter 8

Diastolic Murmurs   63

Learning Objectives   63

Mechanisms of Production   64

Early Diastolic Murmurs   64

Middiastolic Murmurs   64

Late Diastolic Murmurs   65

Pandiastolic Murmurs   65

Clinical Correlation   65

Self-Learning "Unknown" Heart Sounds   67

Self-Learning Questions   67

Answers to Self-Learning "Unknown" Heart Sounds   68

Answers to Self-Learning Questions   68

Chapter 9

Sounds Around S_1 69

Learning Objectives   69

Wide Split S_1 70

Ejection Sounds   70

Midsystolic Clicks   71

Clinical Correlation   72

Self-Learning "Unknown" Heart Sounds   74

Self-Learning Questions   75

Answers to Self-Learning "Unknown" Heart Sounds   75

Answers to Self-Learning Questions   76

Chapter 10

Sounds Around S_2 77

Learning Objectives   77

Paradoxical Split S_2 78

Wide Split S2   78

Fixed Split S2   80

Narrow Split S2   80

Opening Snap   80

Differentiating S3 From the Opening Snap   81

Clinical Correlation   81

Self-Learning "Unknown" Heart Sounds   82

Self-Learning Questions   83

Answers to Self-Learning "Unknown" Heart Sounds   83

Answers to Self-Learning Questions   84

Chapter 11

Friction Rubs—Pericardial and Pleural   85

Learning Objectives   85

Pericardial Friction Rubs   86

Pleural Friction Rubs   87

Clinical Correlation   89

Self-Learning "Unknown" Heart Sounds   90

Self-Learning Questions   90

Answers to Self-Learning "Unknown" Heart Sounds   91

Answers to Self-Learning Questions   91

Bibliography   93

Glossary   95

CHAPTER 1

Introduction

LEARNING OBJECTIVES

After reading this chapter and answering the self-learning questions at the end of the chapter, the learner will be able to do the following:

1. Identify the requirements for adequate cardiac auscultation
2. Differentiate between the use of the bell and diaphragm chest piece of a stethoscope
3. Identify two basic mechanisms of cardiac sound production
4. Identify the four basic characteristics of sound
5. Differentiate between sounds of high-frequency and low-frequency
6. Identify three factors that enter into the transmission of sounds
7. Choose the appropriate area on the chest for auscultation of a selected sound
8. Differentiate between ventricular systole, ventricular diastole, and atrial systole
9. Identify the relationship of cardiac sounds to the cardiac cycle
10. Chart heart sounds using the one through six classification scale

HISTORY

The language of the heart, discerned by cardiac auscultation, is a universal medical language. I was dramatically made aware of this while visiting China. Communications needing no interpretation were those of heart sounds, electrocardiograms, and music. By becoming skillful in listening to and interpreting the language of the heart, you may also join a long line of notable semiologists.

Direct auscultation of the heart was known to Hippocrates (460-377 B.C.), who may have used heart sounds for diagnostic purposes. William Harvey (1578-1657) seems to have been the first to make specific reference to heart sounds. The use of the ear without mechanical aid was the accepted method of listening to the heart until 1816 when Laennec invented the first stethoscope. Rene´ Laennec (1781-1826) by discovering and perfecting the acoustic trumpet became known as the "Father of Auscultation." Laennec named his auscultatory instrument a "stethoscope" from the Greek word meaning "the spy of the chest." His original instrument, which was a hallow wooden cylinder, has been repeatedly revised. These revisions have continued to the present time, making available a great variety of quality stethoscopes.

However perfect the instrument of auscultation, the interpretation of the sounds is still of the essence. Although Laennec devoted his life to the semiology of cardiac auscultation, it was a Czech doctor, Joseph Skoda (1805-1881) who first described the cardiac sounds and murmurs. He pinpointed their localization and defined the clinical auscultatory signs that allowed the diagnosis of cardiac pathology via auscultation. The learner is advised to mimic Skoda and become proficient in pinpointing the location of cardiac sounds and murmurs to arrive at a clinical interpretation of their meaning.

REQUIREMENTS FOR AUSCULTATION

Auscultation must not be performed as an isolated event. The total cardiovascular physical examination includes five important parts: (1) examination of the arterial pulse and blood pressure, (2) inspection of the jugular venous pulse, (3) inspection of the precordium, (4) palpation of the precordium, and (5) auscultation. Each of these parts is important, although only auscultation will be discussed in this book.

One of the first things to consider when undertaking auscultation of the heart is the necessity for the following requirements to be present:

Fig. 1-1. Basic positions for cardiac auscultation. **A**, sitting; **B**, supine; **C**, left lateral recumbent. (Reproduced with permission from L. Caccamo and B. Erickson, *Cardiac Auscultation*, Youngstown, Ohio: St. Elizabeth Hospital Medical Center, 1975.)

1. **Use a quiet, well-lit, warm room.** To facilitate hearing the heart sounds, ambient noise in the room should be eliminated as much as possible. This means that room doors are closed and equipment such as radios and televisions are turned off and conversations stopped. Unfortunately, a quiet room may be one of the hardest elements to achieve. The room needs to be well lit so that the inspection aspect of cardiac examination may be done. Many of the heart sounds can be seen and felt as well as heard. A warm room helps prevent the patient from shivering and causing extraneous sounds underneath the chest piece of the stethoscope.

2. **Have the patient properly disrobed.** The stethoscope should always be placed in direct contact with the chest wall. Most abnormal sounds cannot be heard through clothing because they are lower in frequency and softer than normal heart sounds. Also, listening through clothing will produce sound distortions caused by the stethoscope rubbing against the clothing.

3. **Examine the patient in three positions—supine, sitting, and left lateral recumbent** (Fig. 1-1). Listening in various positions will bring out certain heart sounds, especially some abnormal ones. For instance, the third heart sound (S_3) may be brought out by having the patient turn to the left lateral recumbent position.

4. **Examine the patient from his or her right side.** Being on the patient's right side forces the examiner to reach across the chest to listen to the heart. This stretches out the tubing of the stethoscope and decreases the likelihood of extraneous sounds caused by the tubing hitting objects (e.g., chest wall, side rails).

Fig. 1–2. **A**, *Lightly* applied to skin (no after-imprint is left) transmits *low*-frequency sounds. *B*, Firmly applied to skin (leaves an after-imprint) with skin pulled tautly over the bottom of the bell changes it into a diaphragm and transmits *high*-frequency sounds. (Modified with permission from L. Caccamo and B. Erickson, *Cardiac Auscultation*, Youngstown, Ohio: St. Elizabeth Hospital Medical Center, 1975.)

5. **Use stethoscope with a bell and diaphragm chest piece or one with characteristics of both bell and diaphragm.** Traditionally a stethoscope with both a bell and a diaphragm was essential for complete cardiac auscultation. However, recent technology has provided a stethoscope with only one chestpiece capable of differentiating low-frequency from high-frequency sounds, depending on the pressure applied to the chestpiece. When the chestpiece is used with light pressure, the low-frequency sounds dominate; used with firm pressure the high-frequency sounds are accentuated. Regardless of the technical advances, the traditional principles still apply and therefore will continue to be used in this book.

   a. **Using the bell**

   When the bell is held *lightly* (leaving no after-imprint on the chest), it picks up *low-frequency* sounds.

   Pressure on the bell causes the skin to be pulled tautly over the bottom of the bell, changing the bell to a diaphragm. (Fig. 1-2)

   b. **Using the diaphragm**

   When the diaphragm is applied *firmly* (leaving an after-imprint) it picks up *high-frequency* sounds.

   c. **Differentiating frequencies**

   The frequency of a sound is readily identified by noting with which chest piece of the stethoscope the sound is best heard. A sound best heard, or only heard, with the **bell held lightly is of low frequency**. A sound best heard with the **bell applied firmly, or with a   diaphragm, is of high frequency.** This simple maneuver of listening to a sound with the bell held lightly and

Fig. I–3.   Sites for auscultation: **A**, *left lateral* sternal border (sounds from tricuspid valve and right side of heart heard best); **B**, *apex* (sounds from mitral valve and left side of heart heard best); **C**, *base right* (sounds from aortic valve heard best); **D**, *base left* (sounds from pulmonic valve heard best).

then applied firmly permits you to determine the frequency of the sound to which you are listening. **This is an important point to remember.**

6. **Listen to each area of auscultation.** Listen to each of the following areas, using first the diaphragm and then the bell (Fig. 1-3).
   a. Left lateral sternal border (also known as lower left sternal border [LLSB]): This if the fourth intercostal space (4 ICS) to the left of the sternum. Sounds from the tricuspid valve and right heart are heard best.
   b. Apex: This is the fifth intercostal space (5 ICS) in the mid-clavicular line. Sounds from the mitral valve and left heart are heard best.
   c. Base right (previously known as pulmonic area): This is the second intercostal space (2 ICS) to the right of the sternum. Sounds from the aortic valve are heard best.
   d. Base left (previously known as aortic area): This is the second intercostal space (2 ICS) to the left of the sternum. Sounds from the pulmonic valve are heard best.

7. **Use a sequence for auscultation.** Each time you listen to a heart, begin at the same cardiac area. Listen to all of the above four areas, using the same order each time. This will help you establish a routine for yourself; you will "automatically" listen to all four areas each time you auscultate a heart. The order in which you listen is an individual preference. If you have already established such a personal preference, please do not feel obliged to change it.

8. **Use selective listening.** Listen to one thing at a time. When listening to the first heart sound (S_1), do not be concerned about the second heart sound (S_2). If listening to sounds in systole, do not be concerned about the sounds in diastole. With experience you will be able to rapidly assess the total heart sounds.

Selective listening is a skill that is honed with practice. You may improve this skill by picking out a favorite instrument in a musical arrangement or listening for the ticking of a clock or other repetitive noise in your daily environment. The skill of selective listening is transferable from one situation to another.

Fig. I-4. Time relationships of various cardiac events. From the top down: **A**, left heart pressure curves—aortic, ventricular, and atrial; **B**, heart sounds—normal [S_1, S_2] and extra [S_4, ejection (E), opening snap (OS), and S_3]; **C**, cardiac cycle—ventricular systole and diastole; **D**, electrocardiogram (ECG).

CARDIAC CYCLE

The cardiac cycle consists of two periods: one of contraction (**systole**) and one of relaxation (**diastole**). During **systole** the heart chambers eject blood, and during **diastole** the heart chambers fill with blood. These events are readily represented on pressure curves (Fig.1-4).

Ventricular systole follows closure of the mitral and tricuspid valves. This systolic period is divided into two phases:

1. The first part of the systolic period has two subdivisions.
   a. This period begins with the first initial rise in ventricular pressure after the closure of the mitral and tricuspid valves. It is also known as the **isovolumic contraction phase.**
   b. It is followed by **rapid ventricular ejection,** which occurs when ventricular pressure exceeds the pressure in the aorta and the pulmonary artery. This forces the aortic and pulmonic valves open, causing blood to be rapidly ejected from the ventricles.
2. During the latter part of ventricular systole, ventricular pressure falls, and reduced ventricular ejection occurs. This period lasts until ventricular ejection stops and ventricular diastole begins.

Ventricular diastole follows closure of the aortic and pulmonic valves. This diastolic period is divided into the following three phases.

1. The first third of the diastolic period has two subdivisions:
   a. Initially in this period no blood enters the ventricles; therefore they do not increase in volume. This is also known as the **isovolumic relaxation phase.**
   b. When atrial pressure exceeds ventricular pressure, the mitral and tricuspid valves open, and blood rapidly enters the ventricles. This is also known as the **rapid filling phase.**
2. During the middle third of the diastolic period, there is almost no inflow into the ventricles. This is the period during which both the atrium and the ventricles are relaxed.
3. During the last third of the diastolic period, atrial contraction or "atrial kick" occurs, and the remaining blood is squeezed from the atrium. This is also known as the **late filling phase.**

Atrial systole occurs during the last third of ventricular diastole. Atrial systole may contribute 20% to 25% to ventricular filling. The contribution is less at faster heart rates (100 beats per minute or greater).

CARDIAC SOUND-CYCLE RELATIONSHIP

Cardiac sounds are named according to their sequence of occurrence and are produced at specific points in the cardiac cycle. The initial sound heard is the **first heart sound,** or S_1. It occurs at the beginning of ventricular systole when ventricular volume is maximal. The sound occurring at the end of ventricular systole is the **second heart sound,** or S_2. The period between S_1 and S_2 represents ventricular systole; the period following S_2 and the next S_1 represents ventricular diastole (see Fig. 1-4).

CARDIAC VALVE AREAS

Sounds from the heart valves (mitral, tricuspid, aortic, and pulmonic) are heard at specific areas on the chest.

1. Mitral valve sounds and other left heart sounds are heard best at the apex.
2. Tricuspid valve sounds and other right heart sounds are heard best at the LLSB.
3. Aortic valve sounds are heard best at base right.
4. Pulmonic valve sounds are heard best at base left.

The anatomic location of the valve and the auscultatory area (area heard best) are not synonymous (see Fig. 6-1).

The amount of energy behind the heart sound's production is a contributory factor behind its auscultatory area. Since left heart sounds have more energy behind their productions, they are audible anywhere on the precordium. Right heart sounds, with less energy behind their productions, are usually heard best only at one area—the site to which they radiate.

CARDIAC SOUND PRODUCTION

Cardiac sound production results from at least two basic mechanisms:

1. The sudden acceleration or deceleration of blood, which is mainly influenced by:
   a. The opening and closing of heart valves
   b. Sudden tension of intracardiac structures (chordae tendinae, papillary muscles, or chamber walls)
2. Turbulent blood flow, produced when anatomically there is either
   a. Unilateral protrusion into the bloodstream

b. Circumferential narrowing
c. Flow into a distal chamber of larger diameter than the proximal chamber
d. Flow into a distal chamber of smaller diameter than the proximal chamber
e. High flow rates
f. Abnormal communications (e.g., ventricular septal defects, atrial septal defects)

These conditions can cause eddies in the vascular system and produce vibrations that are audible (Fig. 1-5).

CHARACTERISTICS OF SOUND

Four basic characteristics of sound must be considered: (1) frequency, (2) intensity, (3) quality, and (4) duration.

Fig. 1-5. Factors producing turbulence: **A**, unilateral protrusion into the stream; **B**, circumferential narrowing; **C**, distal chamber larger than proximal one; **D**, distal chamber smaller than proximal one; **E**, high flow rates; **F**, abnormal communications (i.e., VSD).

1. **Frequency** is the number of wave cycles generated per second by a vibrating body. It is vibratory movement of an object in motion that initiates the sound wave cycles that can be discerned by the stethoscope. Frequency determines **pitch,** a subjective sensation that indicates to the listener whether the tone is high or low on a musical scale.
   a. High frequency—the greater the number of wave cycles per second, the higher the frequency and the pitch. High-frequency sounds are best heard with the diaphragm of the stethoscope applied firmly, so that an after-imprint is seen on the chest.
   b. Low frequency—the fewer the number of wave cycles per second, the lower the frequency and pitch. Low-frequency sounds are best heard with the bell of the stethoscope held lightly so that no after-imprint is seen on the chest.
2. **Intensity** is related to the height of the sound wave produced by a vibrating object. Intensity determines the loudness of the perceived sound. High-amplitude waves are produced when an object vibrates with great energy; they are heard as loud sounds. Low-amplitude waves occur when an object vibrates with low energy; they are heard as soft sounds.
3. **Quality** distinguishes two sounds with equal degrees of frequency and intensity, but that come from a different source (piano from violin or heart sounds from breath sounds).
4. **Duration** is the length of time the sound lasts. Heart sounds (S_1 and S_2) are of short duration. Cardiac murmurs or rubs are of long duration.

Each of the above four characteristics should be considered when listening to the heart. Only with experience can the subtleties of sound characteristics be appreciated—much as the quiet stirring of a restless child only awakens its mother while others sleep.

SOUND TRANSMISSION

Three factors enter into how well a sound is transmitted from its source to the auscultator's ears: (1) the type of tissue through which it travels, (2) the quality of the stethoscope, and (3) the human ear.

1. **Types of tissue**
   a. Bone is an excellent transmittor of sound.
   b. Blood and muscle are fair transmittors.

c. Air is a poor transmittor. Therefore the lung, which is normally filled with air, is a poor transmittor of sound. During cardiac auscultation, the heart sounds are heard best in individuals with thin chests because the sounds are being transmitted primarily by blood, muscle, or bone. Cardiac auscultation is more difficult in individuals with thick chests. Obesity, or increased adipose tissue, will decrease sound transmission, as will conditions that cause increased A-P diameter from air-trapping (chronic obstructive lung disease).

2. **Quality of the stethoscope**

   The stethoscope chosen must be of good quality and must have both a bell and a diaphragm chestpiece or one which combines the bell and diaphragm modes into a single-side chestpiece. The quality of the sound transmitted is affected by the design and structural factors of the stethoscope. The tubing of the stethoscope must permit the heart sounds to be transmitted to the ears without loss of quality or the introduction of ambient noises from the environment. Whether to use a scope with a double or single tube is debatable. Theoretically sound transmission is better with the double tube, although there is some difference of opinion on this. The single-tube stethoscope has certain mechanical advantages: less bulk, less ambient noise from the tubes rubbing on each other, and smaller surface to pick up outside noise. The length of the tubing should be as short as feasible for the clinical situation in which it is used routinely. Regardless of the type of stethoscope chosen, the earpieces must fit the examiner's ear canal comfortably; they should be neither too tight nor too loose. Very small ear tips penetrate deeply into the canals, actually causing pain; very large tips may occlude the canals; neither fit facilitates auscultation.

   Amplifying stethoscopes are available, and some clinicians may find them of value. However, in any system with amplification, the heart sounds may be different from the way they are ordinarily heard with the binaural stethoscope. This may cause difficulty in interpreting the sounds and in differentiating the artifact inherent in the instrument from true normal or abnormal heart sounds.

   Regardless of the stethoscope chosen, the most important part is that between the two earpieces. A quality stethoscope in the hands of an individual prepared to use it is an invaluable instrument.

3. **The human ear**

   Individuals differ in their ability to hear. The normal human ear is capable of perceiving sounds with a frequency of 20 to 20,000 cycles/second and a duration of as little as 0.02 seconds. The audible components of heart sounds and murmurs are in the frequency range between 30 to 250 cycles/second. Because of the pecularities of the human ear, high-frequency sounds may seem louder than a low-frequency sound of equal intensity. Also, very loud sounds may momentarily deafen. Therefore the auscultator may have trouble hearing a soft sound that immediately follows a loud sound.

High-frequency perception decreases with age, but this should not interfere with cardiac auscultation because heart sounds are in the lower-frequency range of the hearing capability of the ear. This means that the ability to hear heart sounds should improve with age.

CLASSIFICATION OF SOUNDS AND MURMURS

Sounds and murmurs may be classified on a one through six scale as follows:

1. Not audible during the first few seconds of auscultation; heard after listener tunes in
2. Heard immediately, but faint
3. Loud but without a thrust or thrill
4. Loud with a thrust or thrill
5. Loud with a thrust or thrill and audible with the chestpiece tilted on the chest
6. Loud with a thrust or thrill and audible with chestpiece just off the chest wall

"Thrust" is a *intermittent* palpable (sometimes even visible) sensation at the site being auscultated. This is the sensation felt when palpating the point of maximal impulse at the apex of the heart. "Thrill" is a *continuous* palpable sensation comparable to the vibration felt when a cat purrs.

To chart a sound or murmur, a fraction is used ($^3/_6$ or $^{III}/_{VI}$). The numerator of the fraction indicates where the sound being described fits into the classification system. The demoninator indicates the total number of parts in the classification. Therefore a sound described as a $^3/_6$ would be one that is loud but without a thrust or thrill (as indicated by the numerator "3"). It is being described in a classification system with six parts (as indicated by the denominator "6").

CHARTING HEART SOUNDS

When charting heart sounds, a description of what is heard at each of the four basic auscultatory sites is given. Included in the description are the sound characteristics of frequency, intensity, quality, and duration. In addition, the charting should include:

1. Area of auscultation—LLSB, apex, base right, base left
2. Heart rate
3. Patient's position—e.g., supine, sitting, left lateral recumbent
4. Description of S_1 and S_2
5. Presence of other sounds—splits, ejection sounds, clicks, S_3, S_4
6. Presence of murmurs—noting the following:
   a. Location of valve area where murmur is heard best
   b. Loudness (intensity) by using one through six classification
   c. Frequency (pitch)—low, medium, high
   d. Quality—blowing, harsh, rough, or rumble
   e. Timing—systolic or diastolic
   f. Finer timing—early, mid, or late
   g. Radiation—other locations murmur is heard
   h. Increase or decrease of murmur with respiration, position, special maneuvers, or drugs
7. The type of stethoscope chest piece used—bell or diaphragm
8. The effect of respiration or other maneuvers—inspiration or expiration; e.g., standing, squatting, valsalva

A graphic method of charting heart sounds (the auscultogram) is one of the easiest methods to use. The auscultogram provides an easy means of drawing what is heard during cardiac auscultation. The auscultogram includes the following:

1. A drawing of the chest with the four basic auscultatory sites marked
2. Blank blocks drawn one on top of the other six blocks high; (each block represents one classification in the grading system, one being the bottom block and six being the top block)
3. S_1 and S_2 represented by vertical lines drawn in the blank blocks to indicate the intensity of the sounds
4. S_3, S_4, splits, clicks, and ejection sounds are indicated if heard
5. Murmurs are represented by sine waves:
   a. Widely spaced for low frequency
   b. Close picket fence lines for high frequency

The loudness is represented by the height of the wave on a one through six scale (see Fig. 1-6)

Name _____   Date _____

AUSCULTOGRAM

Indicate the loudness of the S₁ and S₂ at each of the auscultatory sites by drawing vertical lines to the appropriate height in the blank blocks using the one through six scale:

[Each block represents one classification in the grading system.
"1" being the bottom block and "6" being the top block.]

1. Not audible during the first few seconds of auscultation.
2. Heard immediately but faint.
3. Loud but without a *Thrust or Thrill.
4. Loud but with a Thrust or Thrill.
5. Loud with a Thrust or Thrill and audible with the chest piece tilted on the chest.
6. Loud with a Thrust or Thrill and audible with chest piece just off the chest wall.

*"Thrill" is a continuous palpable sensation comparable to the vibration felt when cat purrs.

Draw in extra sound [i.e. S₃, S₄, Ejection (E), or clicks (C)] as indicated.

Draw murmurs in the appropriate cycle.

Use the following sine waves to indicate the frequency/quality:

Use the one through six scale to indicate loudness of murmur by drawing sine wave to height comparable to the loudness of the murmur.

High Frequency = lılıllıllııllıl
(Blowing)

Low Frequency = ᴧᴧᴧᴧᴧ
(Rumbling)

Mixture = ᴧⱵᴧⱵᴧⱵᴧ

Fig. 1–6. An auscultogram, a graphic method of recording heart sounds and murmurs.

MIMICKING SOUNDS

The quality of cardiac sounds can only be captured by the human ear. Phonocardiography produces visual records but not sound. Trying to appreciate heart sounds by looking at a phonocardiogram would be like trying to appreciate a symphony by merely reading the score. The sounds are transcribed, but the music is lost.

A vocabulary that translates the cardiac sounds into spoken syllables has been developed. The normal heart cycle produces a two-sound cadence that can be simulated by the syllables "lub" and "dub." The prefix "l" is used to represent S_1—"lub"; the prefix "d" is used to represent S_2—"dub." Extra sounds such as S_3, S_4, clicks, and snaps are represented by the prefix "b." The intensity of the sounds are represented as follows:

S_1	S_2	Extra sounds
1. Faint sounds-----------"le",	"de",	"be"
2. Normal sounds--------"lub",	"dub",	"bub"
3. Loud sounds-----------"lup",	"dup",	"bup"
4. Very loud sounds-----"lupp",	"dupp",	"bupp"

The cadence for a normal S_4 S_1 S_2 would be mimicked by syllables "bub" "lub" "dub." The cadence for a soft S_4 followed by a normal S_1 S_2 would be vocalized as "be" "lub" "dub"; a normal S_1 and S_2 with a loud S_3 would be vocalized as "lub" "dub" "bupp."

═══   **SELF-LEARNING QUESTIONS**

Select the letter of the correct response or provide requested information. Compare your answers with the answer key at the end of the chapter. Reread the chapter as needed to achieve mastery of the content.

1. Name five of the eight requirements for adequate cardiac auscultation.
   a.
   b.
   c.
   d.
   e.

2. Cardiac sounds and murmurs of low frequency can be best heard by using
   a. a diaphragm chestpiece   **b.** a monaural scope
   c. a bell chestpiece   **d.** either a bell or diaphragm chestpiece

3. The two basic mechanisms of cardiac sound production are
   a.
   b.

4. The number of wave cycles generated per second by a vibrating body is a description of the sound characteristic of
   a. quality   **b.** intensity
   c. frequency   **d.** duration

5. The best type of tissue for transmitting sound is
   a. blood   **b.** fat
   c. air   **d.** bone

6. The frequency perception that is decreased with aging is
   a. low   **b.** medium
   c. high   **d.** none

7. At which area of the chest would mitral or left heart sounds be heard best?
   a. left lateral sternal border   **b.** apex
   c. base right   **d.** base left

8. The rapid filling phase, when the mitral and tricuspid valves open and blood rapidly enters the ventricles, is a part of
   a. atrial systole   **b.** atrial diastole
   c. ventricular systole   **d.** ventricular diastole

9. The cardiac sound that occurs at the beginning of ventricular systole when ventricular volume is maximal is called the
   a. first sound (S_1)   **b.** second sound (S_2)
   c. third sound (S_3)   **d.** fourth sound (S_4)

10. Indicate the graphic representation of a cardiac sound that is loud without a thrill by drawing lines at the appropriate height in the following box:

══ ANSWERS TO SELF-LEARNING QUESTIONS

1. Any five of the following eight responses:
   —A quiet, well-lit, warm room
   —A properly disrobed patient
   —Examine in three positions—supine, sitting, and left lateral recumbent
   —Use a stethoscope with a bell and diaphragm chestpiece
   —Listen to a least four basic areas
   —Use a sequence for auscultation
   —Use selective listening

2. c

3. —The sudden acceleration or deceleration of blood
   —Turbulent blood flow

4. c

5. d

6. a

7. b

8. d

9. a

10.

CHAPTER 2

The First Heart Sound (S₁)

LEARNING OBJECTIVES

After reading this chapter, listening to the accompanying tape, answering the self-learning questions at the end of the chapter, and listening to the "unknowns" on the tape, the learner will be able to do the following:

1. Identify the classical theory behind the production of the S_1
2. Differentiate between a single S_1 and a normal split S_1
3. Recognize a normal S_1 at the various auscultatory sites
4. Identify the physiological factors that affect the intensity of S_1
5. Identify methods of differentiating S_1 from S_2

COMPONENTS OF S$_1$

The **classical** and generally accepted theory for the production of S$_1$ is that S$_1$ is associated with the closure of the mitral (M$_1$) and tricuspid (T$_1$) valves. The **latest** theory indicates that it is the change in the rate of pressure rise in the ventricles, causing sudden tension of intracardiac structures, that contributes to the first heart sound production. Although not entirely true, the classical theory is "simple" and easily correlated with clinical findings and therefore will be used for the text. Since S$_1$ is caused by the closure of two separate valves, both must be considered when listening to it.

M$_1$ is the first audible component of S$_1$. This component normally occurs before T$_1$. (Left-sided mechanical effects occur before right-sided mechanical events.) M$_1$ occurs just after the mitral valve closes. This occurs approximately 0.02 to 0.03 seconds after left ventricular pressure equals left atrial pressure. M$_1$ is of slightly higher intensity and frequency than T$_1$ and is discernible at all the auscultatory sites, but is heard best at the apex. Since it is a high-frequency sound, it is heard best with the diaphragm pressed firmly.

T$_1$ is the second component of S$_1$. It normallly follows M$_1$ just after the tricuspid valve closes. Since there is less energy behind the production of this sound, it may be heard only at left lateral sternal border (LLSB), the area to which T$_1$ radiates or is best heard. Since it is a high-frequency sound, it is heard best with the diaphragm applied firmly.

SPLIT S$_1$

When both components that make S$_1$ (M$_1$ and T$_1$) are separately distinguishable, it is known as a **split.** In a normal split S$_1$, the components making the sound are 0.02 second apart. (Fig. 2-1)

The separation between sounds must be at least 0.02 seconds or greater for the human ear to hear two definite sounds. Since the normal distance between M$_1$ and T$_1$ is *only* 0.02 second, a normally split S$_1$ may be difficult to hear. The ear may perceive it as "slurred" or "fuzzy" and not two separate sounds.

❖   Listen now to an S$_1$ that is split at various distances. The initial split will be 0.08 second—the ear will hear two definite sounds. Gradually the interval of the split decreases—0.06 second; then 0.04 second; then 0.02 second (the duration of the normal split S$_1$). Practice listening until you perceive the difference between a single S$_1$ (only one component audible) and a split S$_1$ (both components audible).

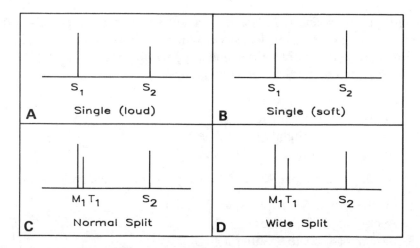

Fig. 2-1. Splitting of the first heart sound (S₁): **A**, single first sound (S₁) louder than the second (S₂); **B**, single S₁ softer than S₂; **C**, normal split first sound (M₁T₁) 0.02 second; **D**, wide split first sound (M₁T₁) 0.04 second. (Reproduced with permission from L. Caccamo and B. Erickson, *Cardiac Auscultation*, Youngstown, Ohio: St. Elizabeth Hospital Medical Center, 1975.)

In a normal heart, the split S_1 may be audible only when listening over the area to which the softer tricuspid component radiates—the LLSB. Although a split S_1 is common in children, it is heard only in about half of normal adults. To be considered a normal split S_1, M_1, and T_1 must be high frequency and heard close together—0.02 second apart. The split is not affected markedly by respiration. When audible, it is heard consistently.

❖ Listen now to a normal S_1 at the various sites.

1. LLSB—split or single S_1 heard
2. Apex—single S_1 heard
3. Base right—Single S_1 heard
4. Base left—single S_1 heard

INTENSITY OF FIRST SOUND (S₁)

The **intensity** or loudness of S_1 also changes, depending on the site auscultated. S_1 is always slightly louder than S_2 at either LLSB or the apex. (The M_1 component of the first sound is heard best at the apex; the T_1 component of the first sound is heard best at the LLSB.) S_1 is softer than the second sound (S_2) at either base left or base right. (The A_1 component of the S_2 is heard best at base right; the P_1 component of S_2 is heard best at base left.)

❖   When a loud sound is followed by a soft sound, the ear perceives the sound as coming **down** a musical scale. When a soft sound is followed by a loud sound, the ear perceives the sound as going **up** a musical scale.

❖   Listen to the normal S_1 at the various sites:

1. LLSB—S_1 slightly louder than S_2
2. Apex—S_1 slightly louder than S_2
3. Base right—S_1 slightly softer than S_2
4. Base left—S_1 slightly softer than S_2

❖ When listening to a normal S_1, the following occurs at each specified site:

1. LLSB—single S_1 or split S_1 louder than S_2
2. Apex—single S_1; louder than S_2
3. Base right—single S_1 softer than S_2
4. Base left—single S_1 softer than S_2

The intensity of S_1 may be affected by the following physiological factors as well:

1. **The anatomy of the chest.** Sounds are easier to hear and therefore louder in patients with thin chests. Sounds are harder to hear and therefore softer in patients with thick chests.
2. **The vigor of ventricular contraction.** Sounds are louder when there is more energy behind their production, as occurs with a tachycardia. Sounds are softer when there is less energy behind their production, as occurs with heart muscle damage (myocardial infarction).
3. **Valve position at the onset of ventricular contraction.** If the valve leaflets are wide open when they are forced closed, as occurs with a short P-R interval, the resulting sound is loud. If the valve leaflets are almost shut when they are forced closed, as occurs with a long P-R interval, the resulting sound is soft.
4. **Pathological alteration of the valve structure** (stiffness of the valve). If the valve orifice is closed and fixed, a loud sound may be heard. If the valve orifice is open and fixed, a soft sound may be heard.

For a synopsis of the physiological factors that vary intensity of S_1 and the resultant type of sound, see Table 2-1.

Table 2-1. Physiological factors that vary first heart sound (S I) intensity

Physiological Factors	Loud S_1	Soft S_1	Variable S_1
1. Anatomy of chest	Thin chest	Emphysema (barrel chest) Obesity Pericardial effusion Edema of chest wall	
2. Vigor of ventricular contraction	Tachycardia: exercise emotion hyperthyroid fever Systemic hypertension	Extensive muscle damage (i.e., myocardial infarction)	
3. Valve position at onset of ventricular contraction when valve mobile	Short PR (except WPW) when valve wide open with wide arc of closure ASD when tricuspid wide open due to volume load	Long PR when valve almost closed with narrow arc of closure	Mobitz I (regular sequential variability of sound.) Atrial fibrillation CHB A—V dissociation (irregular variability of sound)
4. Pathological alteration of the valve structure (STIFF)	Mitral stenosis* which keeps orifice closed and fixed	Mitral regurgitation which keeps valve open and fixed	

*When the first sound is *loud* and the heart rate normal, then *think mitral stenosis.*

(Reproduced with permission from L. Caccamo and B. Erickson, *Cardiac Auscultation,* Youngstown, Ohio: St. Elizabeth Hospital Medical Center, 1975.)

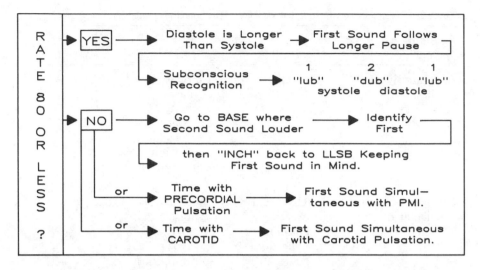

Fig. 2–2. Algorithm for differentiating the first heart sound (S_1) from the second heart sound (S_2). (Reproduced with permission from L. Caccamo and B. Erickson, *Cardiac Auscultation*, Youngstown, Ohio: St. Elizabeth Hospital Medical Center, 1975.)

DIFFERENTIATING S_1 FROM S_2

When listening to the normal heart sounds, S_1 and S_2, it is important to be able to know which sound is the first and which is the second. The following suggestions will help in making this differentiation.

At a heart rate of 80 beats per minute or less, S_1 follows the longer pause. (The time between S_1 and S_2 [systole] is shorter than the time between S_2 and the next S_1 [diastole].) At a heart rate above 80 beats per minute, the diastolic period shortens, becoming equal to systole, and other methods are needed to determine which sound is the first.

In a normal heart, S_2 is always loudest at the base. Therefore listen at the base and determine which of the sounds is the loudest—this is S_2. Then gradually move the stethoscope from the base to the LLSB, keeping in mind which sound is S_1. In this "inching" maneuver, the stethoscope is moved from an area where the sounds are clear to an area where they are not clear. It is a useful technique when multiple or unclear sounds confuse the listener.

Another method of differentiating S_1 from S_2, especially with a rapid heart rate, is to watch your stethoscope while auscultating. The stethoscope may move outward when placed at the point of maximal impulse (PMI), and the sound heard simultaneously with this outward thrust is S_1.

S_1 can also be timed by simultaneously feeling the carotid pulse while listening to the heart. The sound heard when the carotid is felt is S_1. (Peripheral pulses **cannot** be used for timing cardiac sounds because too great of a time lag occurs between ventricular systole and the palpated peripheral pulse.)

A synopsis of the methods of differentiating S_1 from S_2 is depicted in the algorithm of Fig. 2-2.

A big disadvantage of listening to heart sounds from a tape or sound simulator is that the physiological factor (carotid pulse) that aids in sound differentiation is absent. Therefore it may be more difficult to discern the S_1 from S_2. To make it easier for the learner to identify the S_1, the rate of the sounds simulated will be 60 beats per minute unless otherwise indicated.

CLINICAL CORRELATION

After gaining confidence in your ability to identify the first heart sound (S_1), hone your ability by listening to as many real hearts as possible. Listen to the thin and the obese; to adults and children, if possible. Note the similarities and differences. Attempt to distinguish single S_1 from a split S_1. Note the difference in intensity, depending on the site auscultated. Can you differentiate S_1 from S_2 using the physiological factor (carotid pulse) available? Be selective and listen only to the S_1. The other sounds can be ignored for now. Practice recording the S_1 on an auscultogram.

In listening to patients with fever, anemia, aortic insufficiency, or mitral insufficiency, contractility of the heart is increased, and the S_1 will be loud. It will also be loud when the heart is asked to expel blood against increased resistance, as in systemic hypertension. Listen carefully to S_1 in patients with the above findings to see if you can appreciate a louder than normal S_1.

Listen for a soft S_1 in patients with left ventricular dysfunction (myocardial infarction or congestive heart failure). Can you appreciate a soft S_1 in patients with these diagnoses?

═══ SELF-LEARNING "UNKNOWN" HEART SOUNDS

❖ On the tape, listen to the "unknown" heart sounds and identify the sound. Compare your answer with the answer key at the end of the chapter. Relisten to the tape as needed to achieve mastery of the content.

1. Is S_1 single or split?

2. Is S_1 single or split?

3. Is S_1 softer or louder than S_2?

4. Is S_1 softer or louder than S_2?

5. Listen to S_1 at the apex with a bell chestpiece and then with a diaphragm chestpiece.
   Is S_1 normal or abnormal?

═══ SELF-LEARNING QUESTIONS

Select the letter of the correct response. Compare your answers with the answer key at the end of the chapter. Reread the chapter as needed to achieve mastery of the content.

1. The S_1 results from
   a. the opening of the mitral and tricuspid valves
   b. the closure of the mitral and tricuspid valves
   c. the opening of the aortic and pulmonic valves
   d. the closure of the aortic and pulmonic valves

2. The intensity of S_1 would be greater or louder if
   a. the chest wall were enlarged
   b. less vigor were behind ventricular contraction
   c. the P-R interval were short
   d. the mitral valve sacrifice were open and fixed

3. In a normal split S_1, how far apart are the closure sounds?
   a. < 0.0l seconds   b. 0.02-0.03 seconds
   c. 0.03-0.04 seconds   d. > 0.04 seconds

4. The normal split S_1 is best heard at
   a. base right   b. base left
   c. apex   d. LLSB

5. To differentiate S_1 from S_2, which of the following is (are) true?
   (1) At a heart rate of 80 beats per minute or less, S_1 follows the longer pause.
   (2) The S_2 is always loudest at the base.
   (3) With the stethoscope placed on the point of maximal impulse, the sound heard simultaneously with the outward thrust is S_1.
   (4) The sound heard simultaneously with the palpation of the carotid pulse is S_1.

   a. all of the above
   b. 1 and 3 only
   c. 3 and 4 only
   d. 2 and 4 only

ANSWERS TO SELF-LEARNING "UNKNOWN" HEART SOUNDS

1. Single S_1

2. Split S_1

3. Louder S_1

4. Softer S_1

5. Normal S_1 at apex

ANSWERS TO SELF-LEARNING QUESTIONS

1. b

2. c

3. b

4. d

5. a

CHAPTER 3

The Second Heart Sound (S₂)

LEARNING OBJECTIVES

After reading this chapter, listening to the accompanying tape, answering the self-learning questions at the end of the chapter, and listening to the "unknowns" on the tape, the learner will be able to do the following:

1. Identify the classical theory for the production of the S_2
2. Differentiate between a single S_2 and a physiological split S_2 (A_2P_2)
3. Identify the physiology behind the normal physiological splitting of S_2
4. Recognize a normal S_2 at the various auscultatory sites
5. Differentiate between S_1 and S_2 at the various auscultatory sites

Fig. 3–1. Physiological splitting of the second heart sound (S₂). (Reproduced with permission from L. Caccamo and B. Erickson, *Cardiac Auscultation*, Youngstown, Ohio: St. Elizabeth Hospital Medical Center, 1975.)

COMPONENTS OF S$_2$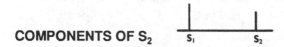

The classical and generally accepted theory for the production of the second heart sound, S_2, is due to the closure of the aortic (A_2) and pulmonic (P_2) valves. Although there is experimental and clinical evidence pointing to other intracardiac factors contributing to the formation of S_2, the "simple" classical theory will be used in this text.

As was true of S_1, the left-sided mechanical event (A_2) has more energy behind its closure and is therefore louder than the right-sided mechanical event (P_2). Also, the left-sided (A_2) normally precedes the right (P_2). The A_2 component is discernible at all the auscultatory sites, but is heard best at base right, the site to which aortic sounds radiate best. It is a high-frequency sound and therefore is heard best with the diaphragm applied firmly.

P_2, the second component making up S_2, is the softer of the two components and is usually only audible at base left, the site to which pulmonic sounds radiate best. It is also a high-frequency sound, and is heard best with the diaphragm applied firmly.

PHYSIOLOGICAL SPLIT S$_2$

If both components that make up S_2 are separately distinguishable, this is known as a **physiological split.** The normal physiological split of S_2 is heard on inspiration; it becomes single on expiration. Thus respiration normally affects the splitting of the S_2 (Fig. 3-1). In the physiological split S_2, A_2 and P_2 are about 0.03 seconds apart. (During inspiration, there is a decrease in intrathoracic pressure that permits an increase in venous return to the right atrium. This increased blood in the right atrium prolongs right ventricular systole and delays pulmonic closing. Since P_2 occurs further from A_2, the split becomes audible.) The respiratory variation of the physiological split is best appreciated during quiet respiration. If expiration is held, a steady state is rapidly reached until the split of S_2 remains fixed somewhere between the width on inspiration and expiration.

As people age, the degree of normal inspiratory splitting of S_2 decreases, so that many older people do not demonstrate audible inspiratory splitting of S_2. The absence of an audible split on inspiration does not indicate pathology, but a distinctly audible splitting of S_2 on expiration is abnormal.

❖   Listen now to a physiological split S_2—split audible on inspiration; sound single on expiration. A split S_2 is normal, or physiological, only if the split occurs during inspiration and becomes single during expiration. It is also normal if the split is not audible. Listen again to an S_2 that is split and an S_2 that is single (only aortic component audible.)

S₂ AUSCULTATORY VARIATIONS

❖   Listen now to the normal S_2 at the various auscultatory sites:

    1.   LLSB—single S_2
    2.   Apex—single S_2
    3.   Base right—single S_2
    4.   Base left—split S_2 on inspiration; single S_2 on expiration

The loudness or intensity of S_2 also changes, depending on the site auscultated. S_2 is always loudest at base right or base left. It is softer than S_1 at LLSB and the apex.

INTENSITY OF S₂

❖   Listen to the loudness of the normal S_2 at the various auscultatory sites:

    1.   LLSB—S_2 softer than S_1
    2.   Apex—S_2 softer than S_1
    3.   Base right—S_2 louder than S_1
    4.   Base left—S_2 louder than S_1

❖   When listening to the normal S_2, the following occurs at each specified site:

1. LLSB—single S_2; S_2 softer than S_1
2. Apex—single S_2; S_2 softer than S_1
3. Base right—single S_2; S_2 louder than S_1
4. Base left—split S_2 on inspiration (A_2P_2); single S_2 on expiration (or always single); S_2 louder than S_1

NORMAL S_1 AND S_2

❖ Review now the normal S_1 and S_2 for each specified site:

	S_1	S_2
LLSB	Single or split; louder	Single; softer
Apex	Single; louder	Single; softer
Base Right	Single; softer	Single; louder
Base Left	Single; softer	Split on inspiration; single on expiration; louder

CLINICAL CORRELATION

When you are confident in your ability to discern S_2, practice it in the clinical area. As you did with S_1, listen to as many different individuals as possible—e.g., young, old, thin, fat. Pay special attention to S_2. Can you identify if S_2 is single or physiologically split? Note the difference in intensity, depending on the site auscultated. Can you differentiate S_2 from S_1? Listen selectively to S_2, but also listen to S_1. Practice recording both S_1 and S_2 on an auscultogram.

Practice hearing the normal physiological split S_2 that **splits on inspiration** and is **single on expiration**. You will hear it at base left. If you do not hear the split, do not think that something is wrong. The physiological split is not audible in everyone, but to be normal the split must **occur on inspiration**.

═══ SELF-LEARNING "UNKNOWN" HEART SOUNDS

❖ On the tape, listen to the "unknown" heart sounds and identify the sound. Compare your answer with the answer key at the end of the chapter. Relisten to the tape as needed to achieve mastery of the content.

1. Is S$_2$ single or physiologically split?

2. Is S$_2$ single or physiologically split?

3. Is S$_1$ or S$_2$ split?

4. Is S$_1$ or S$_2$ split?

5. Listen to S$_2$ at base right with a bell chestpiece and then with a diaphragm chestpiece. Is S$_2$ normal or abnormal?

═══ SELF-LEARNING QUESTIONS

Select the letter of the correct response. Compare your answers with the answer key at the end of the chapter. Reread the chapter as needed to achieve mastery of the content.

1. The normal S$_2$ is produced by
   a. opening of aortic and pulmonic valves
   b. closing of aortic and pulmonic valves
   c. opening of mitral and tricuspid valves
   d. closing of mitral and tricuspid valves

2. The physiological splitting of S$_2$ relates to the fact that during inspiration
   a. closure of the pulmonic valve is delayed
   b. opening of the pulmonic valve is delayed
   c. closure of the aortic valve is delayed
   d. opening of the aortic valve is delayed

3. In the normal heart, when listening at base right, S$_1$ is single; S$_2$ is
   a. split and softer than S$_1$
   b. split and louder than S$_1$
   c. single and softer than S$_1$
   d. single and louder than S$_1$

4. In the normal heart when listening at base left, the physiological splitting of S_2 occurs during
   a. inspiration
   b. expiration
   c. both inspiration and expiration
   d. none of the above

5. In the normal heart, S_2 is louder than S_1 at
   a. left lateral sternal border
   b. apex
   c. base right or left
   d. base left only

ANSWERS TO SELF-LEARNING "UNKNOWN" HEART SOUNDS

1. Single S_2

2. Physiological split S_2

3. Split S_1

4. Split S_2

5. Normal S_2 at base right

ANSWERS TO SELF-LEARNING QUESTIONS

1. b

2. a

3. d

4. a

5. c

CHAPTER 4

Fourth Heart Sound (S$_4$)

LEARNING OBJECTIVES

After reading this chapter, listening to the accompanying tape, answering the self-learning questions at the end of the chapter, and listening to the "unknowns" on the tape, the learner will be able to do the following:

1. Identify the characteristics of S$_4$
2. Identify the physiology behind the production of S$_4$
3. Choose the correct chestpiece of the stethoscope for listening to S$_4$
4. Differentiate right ventricular S$_4$ from left ventricular S$_4$
5. Differentiate a normal split S$_1$ from an S$_4$

NOMENCLATURE OF S₄

The diastolic sound heard just before S_1 is known by the following terms: "fourth heart sound," "atrial gallop," "presystolic gallop," "S_4 gallop," and "S_4." The term "gallop" is used because at a rapid heart rate the presence of the S_4 in the cardiac sequence resembles the canter of a horse. "Atrial gallop" is a misleading term, since the implication is that the atrium is the source of the extra sound when in fact the sound comes from the ventricle(s). S_4 is the most commonly used term.

COMPONENTS OF S₄

S₄ S₁   S₂

S_4 is a low-frequency sound heard just before S_1. Since it is a sound of **low** frequency, it is best heard with the **bell** held lightly. S_4 is a result of decreased ventricular compliance or increased volume of filling. It is a sign of ventricular stress.

S_4 is a diastolic sound that occurs during the late diastolic filling phase (the time at which "atrial kick" occurs). Ventricles receiving this additional blood from the atrium may generate a low frequency vibration—the S_4. This occurs if the ventricles have a decreased compliance or are receiving an increased diastolic volume. An S_4 does not occur unless atrial contraction takes place. Therefore an S_4 is never heard in **atrial fibrillation.**

S_4 may be heard normally in an athletic person under the age of 20 because of the increased diastolic volume that is normal in the young. S_4 also may be indicative of an abnormality of the heart (myocardial infarction is associated with decreased ventricular compliance).

S_4 may be of either left or right ventricular origin. S_4 of left ventricular origin is heard best at the apex during expiration, with the patient in the supine or left lateral position. (Sounds from the left heart radiate best to the apex. Having the patient supine increases the volume of blood in the ventricles, making S_4 louder. Turning the patient to the left lateral position brings the heart closer to the chest, also making S_4 louder.) Common causes of an S_4 of left ventricular origin are severe hypertension, aortic stenosis, primary myocardial disease, coronary artery disease, and cardiomyopathy. S_4 is heard also in conditions with increased cardiac output and stroke volume such as thyrotoxicosis or anemia. Since S_4 is a low-frequency sound, it is best heard with the bell lightly held.

S_4 of right ventricular origin is heard best at the LLSB and is accentuated with inspiration. (Sounds from the right heart radiate best to the LLSB. During inspiration, an increased volume of blood is returned to the right atrium and the right ventricle, making S_4 louder). S_4 may reflect pulmonary valve obstruction, pulmonary stenosis, or pulmonic hypertension. Since S_4 is a low-frequency sound, it is heard best with the bell held lightly.

Dysrhythmias also may affect the presence or absence of S_4. S_4 may be heard when there is a prolonged P-R interval (0.22 seconds or longer) and is commonly heard in first-, second-, or third-degree A-V block. With the prolonged P-R interval, S_4 is not buried in the first sound or heard in conjunction with it. S_4 is never heard in atrial fibrillation, since atrial contraction does not occur in this dysrhythmia.

S_4 is audible with the bell held lightly. (Pressure on the bell causes the skin to be stretched tightly across the bottom of the bell, turning it into a diaphragm.) Thus firm pressure on the bell will cause S_4 to diminish or to disappear.

❖   Listen now to an S_4. Initially only S_1 and S_2 will be heard; then S_4 will be added. Listen to S_4 with the bell held lightly; then to S_4 with the bell applied firmly (note that S_4 disappears).

DIFFERENTIATING S_4 from SPLIT S_1

S_4 M_1T_1 S_2

❖ S_4:

    1. Low frequency before S_1
    2. Heard best with bell lightly held
    3. Pressure on bell causes S_4 to diminish or disappear

Split S_1 (M_1T_1) has the following characteristics:

    1. High frequency
    2. Heard best with diaphragm or bell applied firmly
    3. Sounds 0.02 second apart

S_4 can be decreased by reducing the blood return to the atrium (by standing). S_4 can be increased by increasing atrial blood return (coughing, squatting, or elevating the legs) or by bringing the heart closer to the stethoscope (by rolling the patient to the left lateral decubitus position). If S_4 occurs from the right ventricle, it may become louder with inspiration.

❖   A split S_1 may be increased on standing but is not significantly affected by the other maneuvers. Again listen to a S_4 compared to a split S_1. Listen to a single S_1; then S_1 split; then an S_4 in front of the split S_1. Then to a split S_1 with an S_4 taken in and out.

CLINICAL CORRELATION

Clinical practice in listening to S_4 can be obtained by selecting patients with conditions most likely to have an S_4. Patients with primary myocardial disease, coronary artery disease, cardiomyopathy, aortic stenosis, or severe hypertension may have an S_4 of left ventricular origin that is heard best at the apex. An S_4 of right ventricular origin may be heard in a patient with pulmonary valve obstruction, pulmonary stenosis, or pulmonic hypertension. This S_4 is heard best at the LLSB. Coronary care units are an ideal place to hear an S_4. (Remember that patients with atrial fibrillation can not have S_4). S_4 changes its intensity and distance from S_1 during the various stages of myocardial infarction : (1) initially the S_4 is loud and occurs farther from S_1; (2) as healing occurs and ventricular compliance improves, S_4 becomes softer and closer to S_1 (therefore harder to hear); (3) if the patient has a reinfarction or an extension, S_4 again is loud and occurs farther from S_1. Therefore, in the progression of an uncomplicated myocardial infarction, you would expect S_4 to be initially easy to hear and to gradually become less and less perceptible. Also listen to athletic children who may have an S_4 that is normal. The auscultatory findings between the "normal" S_4 in children and the "pathological" S_4 are similar. The clinical history differentiates the normal S_4 from the pathological S_4. Don't be discouraged if you have difficulty in hearing an S_4 in the clinical area. The S_4 is one of the most difficult sounds to hear, since it is just within the acoustical ability of the ear. To bring out S_4, have the patient do a mild exercise such as coughing or turning to the left side. Turning to the left lateral recumbent position also brings the heart closer to the chest wall and makes S_4 easier to hear. Also listen to S_1 and S_2. Practice recording S_1, S_2, and S_4 on an auscultogram.

═══   SELF-LEARNING "UNKNOWN" HEART SOUNDS

❖ On the tape, listen to the "unknown" heart sounds and identify the sound. Compare your answer with the answer key at the end of the chapter. Relisten to the tape as needed to achieve mastery of the content.

   You are listening to the heart at the LLSB:
      Using the bell held lightly, what do you hear?
      Using the bell applied firmly, what do you hear?
      Using the diaphragm, what do you hear?
1. Is S_1 single or split?
   Is there an S_4?

You are listening to the heart at the LLSB:
   Using the bell held lightly, what do you hear?
   Using the bell applied firmly, what do you hear?
   Using the diaphragm, what do you hear?
2. Is the S_1 single or split?
   Is there an S_4?

You are listening to the heart at the apex:
   Using the bell held lightly, what do you hear?
   Using the bell applied firmly, what do you hear?
   Using the diaphragm, what do you hear?
3. Is S_1 single or split?
   Is there an S_4?

You are listening to the heart at the apex:
   Using the bell held lightly, what do you hear?
   Using the bell applied firmly, what do you hear?
   Using the diaphragm, what do you hear?
4. Is the S_1 single or split?
   Is there an S_4?

You are listening to the heart at the LLSB:
   Using the bell held lightly, what do you hear?
   Using the bell applied firmly, what do you hear?
   Using the diaphragm, what do you hear?
5. When listening with the bell held lightly:
   Is the S_1 single, or split?
   Is there an S_4?

SELF-LEARNING QUESTIONS

Select the letter of the correct response. Compare your answers with the answer key at the end of the chapter. Reread the chapter as needed to achieve mastery of the content.

1. The S_4 is of
   a. low frequency
   c. medium frequency
   b. high frequency
   d. rough frequency

2. S_4 occurs during which phase of the cardiac cycle?
   a. early systolic filling
   c. early diastolic filling
   b. late systolic filling
   d. late diastolic filling

3. You are listening to a patient with atrial fibrillation. You know that an S_4 in this patient is
   a. louder than normal
   b. softer than normal
   c. always heard
   d. never heard

4. Which of the following options would you choose to hear an S_4 best ?
   a. bell firmly pressed
   b. bell lightly held
   c. diaphragm firmly pressed
   d. diaphragm lightly held

5. An S_4 of left ventricular origin would be heard best at
   a. base right
   b. base left
   c. apex
   d. LLSB

=== **ANSWERS TO SELF-LEARNING "UNKNOWN" HEART SOUNDS**

1. Split S_1; no S_4

2. Single S_1; with S_4

3. Single S_1; no S_4

4. Single S_1; with S_4

5. Split S_1; with S_4

=== **ANSWERS TO SELF-LEARNING QUESTIONS**

1. a

2. d

3. d

4. b

5. c

CHAPTER 5

The Third Heart Sound (S₃)

LEARNING OBJECTIVES

After reading this chapter, listening to the accompanying tape, answering the self-learning questions at the end of the chapter, and listening to the "unknowns" on the tape, the learner will be able to do the following:

1. Identify the characteristics of S_3
2. Identify the physiology behind the production of S_3
3. Choose the correct chestpiece of the stethoscope for listening to S_3
4. Differentiate a right ventricular S_3 from a left ventricular S_3
5. Differentiate a physiological split S_2 (A_2P_2) from S_3
6. Differentiate S_3 from S_4

NOMENCLATURE OF S₃

The third heart sound has been known as "ventricular gallop," "protodiastolic gallop," "S₃ gallop," and "S₃." The term "gallop" was used because the sequence of heart sounds with an S₃ or S₄ resembles the canter of a horse, especially when the heart is beating rapidly.

COMPONENTS OF S₃

S₃ is a low-frequency sound heard just after the S₂. Because it is low-frequency, it is heard best with the bell held lightly. S₃ is a result of decreased ventricular compliance or increased ventricular diastolic volume. It may be a sign of ventricular distress, or trouble, as in congestive heart failure. S₃ is a diastolic sound that occurs during the early rapid-filling phase of ventricular filling.

S₃ is normal in children and young adults because they have increased diastolic volumes. Men tend to lose S₃ in their 20s; women lose S₃ in their 30s. An S₃ after the age of 40 is usually associated with cardiac disease except in those individuals physically active in sports. It is heard also in patients with coronary artery disease, cardiomyopathy, incompetent valves, left-to-right shunts (ventricular septal defects or patent ductus arteriosus) and is the **first clinical sign of congestive heart failure.** The preceding conditions may cause a decrease in ventricular compliance, an increase in left ventricular diastolic volume, or both.

S₃ may have its origin in either the right or left ventricle—the latter being more common. Left S₃ is heard best at the apex. (Sounds from the left side of the heart are heard best at the apex because this is the area to which they radiate.) Since S₃ is a low-frequency sound, it is heard best with the bell held lightly.

Right S₃ is heard best at the LLSB or xiphoid area. (Sounds from the right heart are heard best at the LLSB or xiphoid because this is the area to which they radiate).

❖   Listen now to S₃. Initally only S₁ and S₂ will be heard; then S₃ will be added.

DIFFERENTIATING S₃ FROM S₄

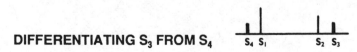

❖ Timing permits S₃ to be distinguished from S₄:

   1. S₃ comes after the S₂
   2. S₄ comes before the S₁

❖   In some individuals both S_3 and S_4 may be present. If the heart rate is normal (60 to 100 beats per minute) and both S_3 and S_4 are present, a **quadruple rhythm** can be heard (four-sound cadence). At a rapid rate S_3 and S_4 may occur simultaneously and are heard as a very loud diastolic sound known as a **summation gallop.** This fusion of S_3 and S_4 occurs because the tachycardia shortens diastole.

For a synopsis of the various sounds that can occur around S_2 and a method of differentiating one from the other, see Table 10-1.

CLINICAL CORRELATION

Clinical practice in listening to S_3 can be obtained by selecting patients with conditions most likely to have an S_3. As was true of S_4, the coronary care unit is one of the best places to hear the pathological S_3. Remember that S_3 is the **first clinical sign of congestive heart failure.** S_3 is normal in children and young adults. The auscultatory findings between the normal S_3 and the pathological S_3 are similar. It is the clinical history that differentiates the two sounds. S_3 is easier to hear than S_4, but you may still need to make S_3 more perceptible by having the patient do a mild exercise such as coughing or turning to the left side. Changing the patient's position from sitting to supine may also bring out S_3. (This is also true of S_4) Having the patient grip one hand with the other may also bring out an S_3 (or S_4). The hand grip increases peripheral vascular resistance, blood pressure, heart rate, and cardiac output. Also listen to S_1, S_2, and S_4. Can you differentiate the split S_1 from an S_4; the physiological split S_2 from S_3; S_4 from S_3? Practice recording the S_1, S_2, S_3, and S_4 on an auscultogram.

══ SELF-LEARNING "UNKNOWN" HEART SOUNDS

❖ On the tape, listen to the "unknown" heart sounds and identify the sound. Compare your answer with the answer key at the end of the chapter. Relisten to the tape as needed to achieve mastery of the content.

You are listening to the heart at the apex:
Using the bell held lightly, what do you hear?
Using the bell applied firmly, what do you hear?
Using the diaphragm, what do you hear?
1. Is S_2 single, split, or is there an S_3?

You are listening to the heart at the base left:
    Using the bell held lightly, what do you hear?
    Using the bell applied firmly, what do you hear?
    Using the diaphragm, what do you hear?
2. Is S_2 single, split, or is there an S_3?

You are listening to the heart at the apex:
    Using the bell held lightly, what do you hear?
    Using the bell applied firmly, what do you hear?
    Using the diaphragm, what do you hear?
3. Is there an S_4 or an S_3?

You are listening to the heart at the apex:
    Using the bell held lightly, what do you hear?
    Using the bell applied firmly, what do you hear?
    Using the diaphragm, what do you hear?
4. Is there an S_4 or a S_3?

You are listening to the heart at the apex:
    Using the bell held lightly, what do you hear?
    Using the bell applied firmly, what do you hear?
    Using the diaphragm, what do you hear?
5. Is there an S_4 or an S_3?

≡≡≡ SELF-LEARNING QUESTIONS

Select the letter of the correct response. Compare your answers with the answer key at the end of the chapter. Reread the chapter as needed to achieve mastery of the content.

1. S_3 is a low-frequency sound that is heard best with which chestpiece of the stethoscope?
   a. bell held lightly   **b.** bell applied firmly
   c. diaphragm held lightly   **d.** diaphragm applied firmly

2. S_3 is the result of _____ ventricular compliance or _____ ventricular diastolic volume.
   a. increased; increased   **b.** decreased; increased
   c. increased; decreased   **d.** decreased; decreased

3. S_3 is heard in an 8-year-old boy with no other abnormal clinical findings. You consider the third heart sound to be
   a abnormal, needing consultation   **b.** abnormal, watch closely
   c. never normal   **d.** normal in children

4. S_3 of left ventricular origin would be best heard at
   a. base right
   b. base left
   c. apex
   d. left lateral sternal border

5. The first clinical sign of congestive heart failure is
   a. S_4
   b. wide split S_1
   c. S_3
   d. wide split S_2

ANSWERS TO SELF-LEARNING "UNKNOWN" HEART SOUNDS

1. Single S_2 with S_3

2. Physiological split S_2

3. S_4

4. S_3

5. S_4 and S_3

ANSWERS TO SELF-LEARNING QUESTIONS

1. a

2. b

3. d

4. c

5. c

CHAPTER 6

Murmurs—General Information

LEARNING OBJECTIVES

After reading this chapter, listening to the accompanying tape, answering the self-learning questions at the end of the chapter, and listening to the "unknowns" on the tape, the learner will be able to do the following:

1. Define a murmur
2. Identify the common causes of murmurs
3. Identify the six characteristics to be considered in murmur identification
4. Differentiate between murmurs of high, medium, and low frequency
5. Differentiate between murmurs having the quality of "blow," "harsh," "rough," or "rumble"
6. Differentiate between systolic and diastolic murmurs

CHARACTERISTICS OF MURMURS

Murmurs are defined as sustained noises that are audible during the time periods of systole, diastole, or both.

Common causes of murmurs include backward regurgitation (a leaking valve, septal defect, or arteriovenous connection); forward flow through narrowed or deformed valve; a high rate of blood flow through normal or abnormal valves; vibration of loose structures within the heart (chordae tendineae); and continuous flow through A-V shunts.

To identify a murmur, there are six characteristics that you need to consider:

1. Location—valve area where murmur heard best
2. Loudness (intensity)—use the one to six grading system
3. Frequency (pitch)—i.e., low, medium, high
4. Quality—blowing, harsh, rough, or rumble
5. Timing—-systolic or diastolic
6. Radiation—where else murmur heard

Location of Murmurs

The **location of murmurs,** as with normal heart sounds, originates near a heart valve. You will find it necessary to listen to the four basic areas previously discussed, plus a fifth area, commonly called Erb's Point, which is located at the third intercostal space along the LLSB (Fig. 6-1).

To determine murmur location, listen to all of the basic areas and decide at which area the murmur is heard best. You will find that murmurs from certain valves tend to be heard best "downstream" from the valve as follows:

Valve	Heard Best
1. Mitral	Apex
2. Tricuspid	LLSB
3. Pulmonic	Base left
4. Aortic (systolic)	Base right
Aortic (diastolic)	Erb's point

Loudness of Murmurs

Loudness (intensity) is judged by using the same one through six classification previously discussed for heart sounds. The loudness of the murmur should not be thought to correlate with its significance. Some

Fig. 6–1. Valve areas: *Anatomic* area is represented by solid bars. M = mitral valve; T = tricuspid valve; A = aortic valve; P = pulmonic valve. *Auscultatory* areas (areas where sound is heard best) are represented by arrows. Star ($\star$) represents Erb's point.

insignificant abnormalities may have loud murmurs; whereas the same abnormality that has progressed in significance may be softer. (Think of a plaque occluding an artery. Minimal plaque may have intense sustained noise [bruit]; complete occlusion may have no sound.)

Frequency of Murmurs

Frequency (pitch) indicates whether the sound heard is high, medium, or low. This is easily determined, since murmurs of high frequency are best heard with the diaphragm chestpiece; those of low frequency with the bell held lightly; and those of medium frequency with either bell or diaphragm chestpiece. With practice, the frequency of the murmur will alert you to the presence of a specific abnormality (Table 6-1).

❖ Listen now to murmurs that are considered high, medium, and low.

Quality of Murmurs

Quality is closely related to frequency and is described as "blowing" (mainly high frequency); "harsh" or "rough" (medium frequency—mix of high and low frequencies); and "rumble" (mainly low frequency). The quality of the murmur alerts the astute clinician to the presence of a specific abnormality, see Table 6-1.

❖ Listen now to murmurs that are described as "blowing," "harsh" or "rough," and "rumble." For a differentiation of the common murmurs by frequency and quality, see Table 6-1.

Timing of Murmurs

Timing means that you can identify whether the sustained noise is occurring between S_1 and S_2—a systolic murmur; or between S_2 and S_1—a diastolic murmur. In some abnormalities the murmur will be heard both in systole and diastole.

❖ Listen now to a heart rate of 60 beats per minute. First, a systolic blow murmur will be added, then removed. Then a diastolic rumble murmur will be added and removed. Murmurs of different frequency and quality have been deliberately selected to help you tell the difference between systole and diastole.

As a beginning auscultator, you may not be able to pinpoint the timing any more precisely than to determine if the murmur occurs in systole or diastole. However, with experience you'll note that even **"finer timing"** (early, mid, late, or pan) is possible. A murmur is said to be "early" if its peak intensity occurs early in the cycle; "mid" if the peak intensity occurs in the middle of the cycle; and "late" if the peak intensity occurs late in the cycle. If the murmur is heard throughout the cycle with equal intensity, it is known as a "pan or holo" murmur.

❖ Listen now to a heart rate of 60 beats per minute. Then a murmur will be added in the systolic period: early, mid, late, and pan.

❖ Listen now to a heart rate of 60 beats per minute. Then a murmur will be added in the diastolic period: early, mid, late, and pan.

Table 6-1. Differentiation of common cardiac abnormalities by pitch and quality

Pitch	Frequency (cycles/sec)	Quality	Abnormality	Chest Piece
High	200–400	Blowing	Mitral regurgitation Tricuspid regurgitation Aortic regurgitation VSD	Diaphragm
Medium	100–200	Harsh	Aortic stenosis	Either
		Rough	Pulmonic regurgitation ASD Increase flow of pulmonary outflow tract	Bell
Low	< 100	Rumble	Mitral stenosis	Bell

Modified with permission from L. Caccamo and B. Erickson, *Cardiac Auscultation*, (Youngstown, Ohio: St. Elizabeth Hospital Medical Center, 1975.)

Radiation of Murmurs

Radiation of the murmur is assessed when you determine in what other areas the sound is audible in addition to where you heard it best. Each cardiac abnormality has a classical radiation. See Figs. 7-1 and 8-1 for the radiation patterns of common cardiac abnormalities.

Shape of Murmurs

Murmurs have an identifiable **shape** to their sound that is often described in musical terminology. A "crescendo/decrescendo" (diamond-shaped) murmur starts softly, peaks in intensity, then diminishes (systolic murmur of aortic stenosis). A "decrescendo" murmur begins loud and gets progressively quieter (diastolic murmur of aortic regurgitation). A "pan or holo" murmur remains unchanged from the onset to the end of the sound (pansystolic murmur of severe mitral regurgitation). A "crescendo" murmur starts out soft and becomes progressively louder (late systolic murmur of mitral valve prolapse). A "decrescendo/ crescendo" murmur starts out loud, gets softer, then becomes loud again (diastolic murmur of mitral stenosis).

Special Maneuvers

Special maneuvers to help in differentiation of one murmur (or sound) from another include valsalva, exercise, respiration, hand grip, and the use of amyl nitrate. The **valsalva** is performed by asking the patient to bear down or strain. This manuever increases intrathoracic pressure and decreases venous return to the right heart. Most murmurs decrease during the strain phase of the valsalva. After release of the straining phase, right-sided events return in 1 to 3 beats, whereas left-sided events return in 4 to 11 beats. **Exercise** increases the heart rate and thereby increases blood flow; murmurs (and sounds) may be *increased* in intensity. **Respiration** also changes the loudness of sounds by bringing the heart closer to the chest wall and making the heart sounds louder. Therefore faint diastolic murmurs of aortic or pulmonic regurgitation may be heard better during *expiration*. [Note: This is not to be confused with the physiological effects of respiration. During inspiration, right-sided cardiac events are louder due to the increased venous return.] **Hand grip** in which one hand is gripped with the other causes an increased peripheral vascular resistance, blood pressure, heart rate, and cardiac output. This maneuver increases left-sided regurgitant murmurs (aortic and mitral regurgitation and ventricular septal defect) and causes left-sided ejections murmurs to decrease (aortic stenosis). **Amyl nitrate** causes a decreased peripheral vascular resistance and increase in heart rate and in venous return. Following inhalation of amyl nitrate, *forward flow murmurs* (aortic stenosis, mitral stenosis, pulmonic stenosis, and tricuspid stenosis) *increase*; *left-sided regurgitant murmurs* (aortic regurgitation and mitral regurgitation) become *softer*.

===== **SELF-LEARNING "UNKNOWN" HEART SOUNDS**

❖ On the tape, listen to the "unknown" heart sounds and identify the sound. Compare your answer with the answer key at the end of the chapter. Relisten to the tape as needed to achieve mastery of the content.
Determine the frequency of the following sustained sounds:

1. This sound is heard best with the diaphragm applied firmly.

2. This sound is heard equally well with either the bell or the diaphragm.

3. This sound is heard best with the bell held lightly.
   Determine the quality of the following sounds:

4. This sound is heard best with the diaphragm applied firmly.

5. This sound is heard best with the bell held lightly.

===== **SELF-LEARNING QUESTIONS**

Select the letter of the correct response or provide requested information. Compare your answers with the answer key at the end of the chapter. Reread the chapter as needed to achieve mastery of the content.

1. A sustained noise that is audible during the time period of systole, diastole, or both periods is descriptive of
   a. systolic murmur   **b.** diastolic murmur
   c. murmur   **d.** blow

2. Name two common causes for murmur production.
   a.
   b.

3. Name the six characteristics you need to consider to identify a murmur.
   a.
   b.
   c.
   d.
   e.
   f.

4. If the sustained noise occurs between S_1 and S_2, the murmur is called:
   a. systolic
   b. diastolic
   c. regurgitant
   d. ejection

ANSWERS TO SELF-LEARNING "UNKNOWN" HEART SOUNDS

1. High frequency

2. Medium frequency

3. Low frequency

4. Blow

5. Rumble

ANSWERS TO SELF-LEARNING QUESTIONS

1. c

2. Any two of the following:

   —Backward regurgitation
   —Forward flow through narrow or deformed valve
   —High rate of blood flow thru normal or abnormal valve
   —Vibration of loose structures within the heart

3. —Location
   —Loudness
   —Frequency
   —Quality
   —Timing
   —Radiation

4. a

CHAPTER 7

Systolic Murmurs

LEARNING OBJECTIVES

After reading this chapter, listening to the accompanying tape, answering the self-learning questions at the end of the chapter, and listening to the "unknowns" on the tape, the learner will be able to do the following:

1. Define systolic murmur
2. Identify the mechanism(s) of systolic murmur production
3. Identify the characteristics of an early systolic, midsystolic, late systolic, and pansystolic murmur
4. Differentiate between an early systolic, midsystolic, late systolic, and pansystolic murmur
5. Identify common adult abnormalities having systolic murmurs

Systolic murmurs are sustained noises that are audible between S_1 and S_2. In some patients systolic murmurs may be normal. This may be true of babies or children because of their thin chest walls. In adults a "normal" systolic murmur may be the result of increased blood flow, as in pregnancy. A systolic murmur would probably be heard in most normal hearts if listened for in a sound proof room.

MECHANISM OF SYSTOLIC MURMUR PRODUCTION

Systolic murmurs occur during the ventricular systolic period. Forward flow across the aortic or pulmonic valves or regurgitant flow from the mitral or tricuspid valve may produce a systolic murmur. The valves may be normal (but with a high rate of flow) or abnormal. Systolic murmurs may be heard in the normal hearts of children or pregnant women. Common abnormalities having a systolic murmur include mitral insufficiency, tricuspid insufficiency, aortic stenosis, pulmonic stenosis, and interventricular septal defects.

EARLY SYSTOLIC MURMURS

An **early systolic murmur** begins with S_1 and peaks in the first third of systole. It may be caused by a modified regurgitant murmur with backward flow through an incompetent valve, a septal defect, or an A-V communication. Common causes are a small ventricular septal defect or the innocent murmurs of children.

❖   Listen now to a heart rate of 60 beats per minute. Then an early systolic murmur will be added.

An **innocent systolic** murmur is usually either **early** or **ejection** (see midsystolic murmurs). Its grade is a $^2/_6$ or less. It is common in children. This sound is considered normal or "innocent" if there is no recognizable heart lesion and if:

1. Normal split S_2 is heard (S_2 splits on inspiration; single on expiration)
2. Normal jugular venous and carotid pulses are present
3. Normal precordial pulsation is present
4. Normal history, chest x-ray, and ECG exist

Common causes are:

1. Pulmonary outflow tract murmur (ejection)

2. Vibratory (humming or musical) that are heard in children (ages 2 to 7) at LLSB

Innocent systolic murmurs may also be heard in the elderly, most frequently due to sclerotic changes of the aortic valve. The murmur is usually of short duration, faint with a grade of $^2/_6$ or less. The innocent murmur of the elderly may continue a benign course for years or gradually progress and cause symptoms. Other causes of **innocent systolic murmurs** include conditions in which there is increased blood flow such as hyperthyroidism, anemia, fever, exercise, and pregnancy (92%).

❖   Listen now to a heart rate of 60 beats per minute. An early innocent murmur will be added. The early systolic murmur will be compared to a midsystolic murmur.

MIDSYSTOLIC MURMURS

A **midsystolic murmur** begins shortly after the first sound (S_1), peaks in midsystole, and does not quite extend to S_2. It is known as an "ejection" murmur. It is a crescendo-decrescendo murmur ("diamond shaped") that builds up and decreases symmetrically. It may be caused by forward blood flow through a narrow or irregular valve such as found in aortic or pulmonic stenosis.

❖   Listen now to a heart rate of 60 beats per minute. A midsystolic murmur will be added, which is medium in frequency and harsh in quality.

LATE SYSTOLIC MURMURS

A **late systolic murmur** begins in the latter one half of systole, peaks in the later third of systole, and extends to S_2. It is a modified regurgitant murmur with a backward flow through an incompetent valve. It is commonly heard in papillary muscle disorders and in the mitral valve prolapse syndrome.

❖   Listen now to a heart rate of 60 beats per minute. A late systolic murmur will be added that is high in frequency and blowing in quality.

PANSYSTOLIC (OR HOLOSYSTOLIC) MURMUR

A **pansystolic (or holosystolic) murmur** is heard continuously throughout systole. It begins with the S_1 and ends with S_2. Since the pressure remains higher throughout systole in the ejecting chamber than the receiving

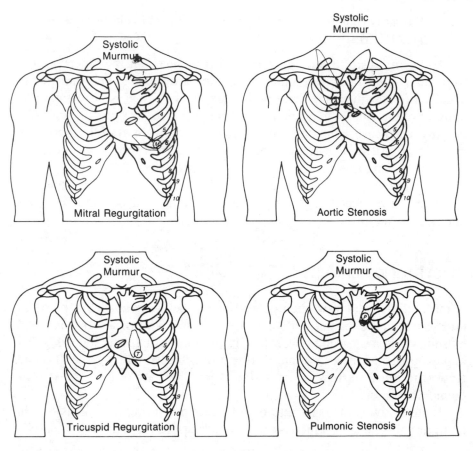

Fig. 7-1. Common cardiac abnormalities with systolic murmur(s): area where murmur is heard best is *circled*; area of usual radiation is *shaded*.

chamber, the murmur is continuous. It is heard commonly in mitral regurgitation, tricuspid regurgitation, and ventricular septal defect.

❖   Listen now to a heart rate of 60 beats per minute. Then a pansystolic (holosystolic) murmur will be added that is of high-frequency and blowing in quality.

A review of the common adult abnormalities having systolic murmurs is provided in Fig. 7-1.

CLINICAL CORRELATION

One of the easiest ways of gaining clinical practice in listening to systolic murmurs is to seek out patients in whom these murmurs have already been identified. Common pathologies having this type of murmur are mitral regurgitation, tricuspid regurgitation, aortic stenosis, or pulmonic stenosis. Patients with mitral valve prolapse may have a late systolic murmur. Systolic murmurs may also be heard in normal hearts, as in the innocent murmur of childhood or pregnancy. Initially try to determine whether the murmur is in systole or in diastole. With practice you will be able to tell if it is early, mid, or late in systole. Also determine the following: (1) location—valve area where heard best, (2) loudness, (3) frequency, (4) quality, and (5) radiation. Practice recording the systolic murmur on an auscultogram. Also practice writing a narrative description of the systolic murmur heard.

Keep in mind that murmurs originating on the right side of the heart generally *increase with inspiration* and that those from the left side *decrease.* You may also which to try some of the manuevers decribed under **Special maneuver** section in Chapter 6.

===== **SELF-LEARNING "UNKNOWN" HEART SOUNDS**

❖ On the tape, listen to the "unknown" heart sounds and identify the sound. Compare your answers with the answer key at the end of the chapter. Relisten to the tape as needed to achieve mastery of the content.
Listen to the following systolic murmurs.

1. Is the murmur early systolic, midsystolic, late systolic, or pansystolic in nature?

2. Is the murmur early systolic, midsystolic, late systolic, or pansystolic in nature?

3. Is the murmur early systolic, midsystolic, late systolic, or pansystolic in nature?

4. Is the murmur early systolic, midsystolic, late systolic, or pansystolic in nature?

5. Is the quality of this late systolic murmur a "blow" or a "rumble?"

SELF-LEARNING QUESTIONS
=====

Select the letter of the correct response. Compare your answers with the answer key at the end of the chapter. Reread the chapter as needed to achieve mastery of the content.

1. Sustained noises that are audible between the S_1 and S_2 are descriptive of
    a. systolic murmur   **b.** diastolic murmur
    b. ejection sound   **d.** friction rubs

2. Regurgitant blood flow across which valves will cause a systolic murmur?
   a. mitral and aortic   **b.** mitral and tricuspid
   c. tricuspid and pulmonic   **d.** pulmonic and aortic

3. Forward blood flow across which abnormal valves will cause a systolic murmur?
   a. mitral and aortic   **b.** mitral and tricuspid
   c. tricuspid and pulmonic   **d.** pulmonic and aortic

4. Common adult abnormalities having a systolic murmur include
   a. mitral insufficiency and aortic insufficiency
   b. mitral stenosis and aortic insufficiency
   c. mitral insufficiency and aortic stenosis
   d. mitral stenosis and aortic stenosis

5. A murmur that begins shortly after S_1, peaks in mid-systole, and does not quite extend to S_2 is descriptive of a(n)
   a. early systolic murmur   **b.** midsystolic murmur
   c. late systolic murmur   **d.** pansystolic murmur

ANSWERS TO SELF-LEARNING "UNKNOWN" HEART SOUNDS

1. Early systolic murmur

2. Midsystolic murmur

3. Pansystolic murmur

4. Late systolic murmur

5. Blow quality

ANSWERS TO SELF-LEARNING QUESTIONS

1. a

2. b

3. d

4. c

5. b

CHAPTER 8

Diastolic Murmurs

LEARNING OBJECTIVES

After reading this chapter, listening to the accompanying tape, answering the self-learning questions at the end of the chapter, and listening to the "unknowns" on the tape, the learner will be able to do the following:

1. Define a diastolic murmur
2. Identify the mechanisms of a diastolic murmur production
3. Identify the characteristics of an early diastolic, middiastolic, late diastolic, and pandiastolic murmur
4. Differentiate between an early diastolic, middiastolic, late diastolic, and pandiastolic murmur
5. Identify common adult abnormalites having diastolic murmur(s)
6. Differentiate between systolic and diastolic murmurs

Diastolic murmurs are sustained noises that are audible between S₂ and the next S₁. Unlike systolic murmurs, diastolic murmurs should usually be considered pathological and **not** normal.

MECHANISMS OF PRODUCTION

There are three main **mechanisms of diastolic murmur** production:

1. **Aortic or pulmonic valve incompetence.** During ventricular diastole, the pressure in the ventricles is less than that in the aorta or the pulmonary artery. If the aortic or pulmonic valves are incompetent, blood regurgitates back into the ventricles. The sustained noise of this regurgitation is the diastolic murmur.
2. **Mitral stenosis or tricuspid stenosis.** During the rapid filling phase of ventricular diastole, if the blood is forced into the ventricles through stenotic valves, a diastolic murmur occurs.
3. **Increased blood flow across mitral or tricuspid valves.** If there is an increase in volume or velocity of blood flow across the mitral valve or tricuspid valve during ventricular diastole, a diastolic murmur occurs.

EARLY DIASTOLIC MURMURS

An **early diastolic murmur** begins with the S₂ and peaks in the first third of diastole. This makes S₂ difficult to hear, whereas S₁ is easily heard. It is usually a regurgitant murmur with backward flow through an incompetent valve. Common causes are aortic regurgitation and pulmonic regurgitation.

❖   Listen now to a heart rate of 60 beats per minute. An early diastolic murmur will be added that is high in frequency and blowing in quality.

MIDDIASTOLIC MURMURS

A **middiastolic murmur** begins after the S₂ and peaks in middiastole. (Both S₂ and S₁ are heard clearly.) Common causes are mitral stenosis and tricuspid stenosis. The murmur is low in frequency and rumbling in quality.

❖   Listen now to a heart rate of 60 beats per minute. A middiastolic murmur will be added that is low in frequency and rumbling in quality.

LATE DIASTOLIC MURMURS

A **late diastolic murmur** begins in the latter one half of diastole, peaks in the later third of diastole, and extends to S_1. (S_2 is heard clearly; S_1 is difficult to hear). It is also known as **presystolic** murmur. It is commonly a component of the murmur of mitral stenosis or tricuspid stenosis. This murmur is low in frequency and rumbling in quality.

❖　　Listen now to a heart rate of 60 beats per minute. A late diastolic murmur will be added that is low in frequency and rumbling in quality. Listen next to a heart rate of 60 beats per minute. A mid-diastolic and a late diastolic murmur will be added that are low in frequency and rumbling in quality.

PANDIASTOLIC MURMURS

A **pandiastolic murmur** begins with S_2 and extends throughout the diastolic period. (Both S_2 and S_1 are difficult to hear.) Patent ductus arteriosus, the prototype of aorticopulmonary connections, is a classical example of this murmur. This condition is unusual in an adult, since it is usually corrected in childhood. It is usually heard best at base left and has both a systolic and diastolic component. It is therefore known as a continuous murmur. It may be best heard with the bell chestpiece.

❖　　Listen next to a heart rate of 60 beats per minute. A pandiastolic murmur will be added that is low in frequency.

❖　　Finally, listen to a typical murmur of patent ductus arteriosus with both systolic and diastolic components.

For a review of the common adult abnormalities having diastolic murmurs see Fig. 8-1.

CLINICAL CORRELATION

To gain skill in listening to diastolic murmurs, seek out patients in whom these murmurs have already been identified. Common pathologies having this type of murmur are mitral stenosis, tricuspid stenosis, aortic regurgitaion, and pulmonic regurgitation. Initially try to determine whether the murmur is in diastole or in systole. Also determine the following: (1) location, (2) loudness, (3) frequency, (4) quality, and (5) radiation. Practice differentiating systolic from diastolic murmurs. Also practice recording the diastolic murmur on an auscultogram. In addition, write a narrative description of the diastolic murmur heard.

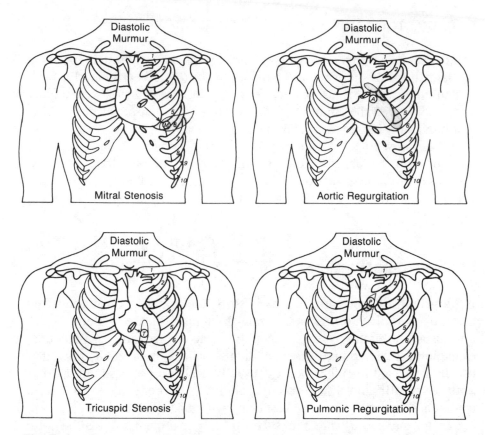

Fig. 8–1. Common cardiac abnormalities with diastolic murmur(s): area where murmur is heard best is *circled*; area of usual radiation is *shaded*.

In a patient with a murmur of mitral stenosis, you may be able to hear the murmur by first finding the point of maximal impulse. Mark the PMI with a finger and then place bell of stethoscope lightly over this area. The typical rumble of mitral stenosis may be heard. It may be inaudible when the stethoscope is moved out of this spot. The murmur can be brought out by having the patient cough several times (a mild exercise) or simply by the exertion from having the patient turn to the left lateral position. (S_3 from the left ventricle may also be heard at this identical point and by using the same maneuvers).

Some aortic diastolic murmurs may be heard along the right sternal border (third and fourth ICS). The development of aortic regurgitation with the murmur along the right sternal border (normally heard at Erb's point on left sternal border) in a patient with a preexistent *diastolic* hypertension may be an indication of aortic aneurysm or dissection, or both.

=== **SELF-LEARNING "UNKNOWN" HEART SOUNDS**

❖ On the tape, listen to the "unknown" heart sounds and identify the sound. Compare your answers with the answer key at the end of the chapter. Relisten to the tape as needed to achieve mastery of the content.

Listen to the following diastolic murmurs.

1. Is the murmur early diastolic, middiastolic, late diastolic, or pandiastolic in nature?

2. Is the murmur early diastolic, middiastolic, late diastolic, or pandiastolic in nature?

3. Is the murmur early diastolic, middiastolic, late diastolic, or pandiastolic in nature?

4. Is the murmur early diastolic, middiastolic, late diastolic, or pandiastolic in nature?

5. What is the quality of this middiastolic murmur?

=== **SELF-LEARNING QUESTIONS**

Select the letter of the correct response. Compare your answers with the answer key at the end of the chapter. Reread the chapter as needed to achieve mastery of the content.

1. Sustained noises that are audible between S_2 and S_1 are
   a. systolic murmur   b. diastolic murmur
   c. ejection sound   d. friction rub

2. Regurgitant blood flow across which valves will cause a diastolic murmur?
   a. mitral and aortic   b. mitral and tricuspid
   c. tricuspid and pulmonic   d. pulmonic and aortic

3. Forward blood flow across which abnormal valves will cause a diastolic murmur?
   a. mitral and aortic   b. mitral and tricuspid
   c. tricuspid and pulmonic   d. pulmonic and aortic

4. Common adult abnormalities having a diastolic murmur include
   a. mitral stenosis and aortic insufficiency
   b. mitral stenosis and aortic stenosis
   c. mitral insufficiency and aortic insufficiency
   d. mitral insufficiency and aortic stenosis

5. A murmur that begins with S_2 and peaks in the first third of diastole is a(n)
   a. early diastolic murmur   b. middiastolic murmur
   c late diastolic murmur   d. pandiastolic murmur

ANSWERS TO SELF-LEARNING "UNKNOWN" HEART SOUNDS

1. Middiastolic murmur

2. Early diastolic murmur

3. Late diastolic murmur

4. Pandiastolic murmur

5. "Rumble" quality

ANSWERS TO SELF-LEARNING QUESTIONS

1. b

2. d

3. b

4. a

5. a

CHAPTER 9

Sounds Around S_1

LEARNING OBJECTIVES

After reading this chapter, listening to the accompanying tape, answering the self-learning questions at the end of the chapter, and listening to the "unknowns" on the tape, the learner will be able to do the following:

1. Differentiate a normal split S_1 ($M_1 T_1$) from a wide split $S_1 (M_1 \, T_1)$
2. Differentiate a pulmonic from an aortic ejection sound
3. Identify the characteristics of a midsystolic click
4. Identify the following:
   a. normal split S_1
   b. wide split S_1
   c. ejection sound—aortic or pulmonic
   d. midsystolic click
   e. S_4

WIDE SPLIT S₁   M₁ T₁   S₂

An abnormal split S_1 may result from either electrical or mechanical causes. The resulting asynchrony of the ventricles causes the mitral and tricuspid valve closure sounds to be a duration of 0.04 to 0.05 second apart compared to the normal split S_1 of 0.02 second. The resulting sound is known as a wide split S_1. The wide split S_1 results when the physiological split is augmented by conditions that delay pulmonic closure. Electrical causes include conduction problems such as right bundle branch block, ventricular premature beats (especially left), ventricular tachycardia, third-degree heart block with idioventricular rhythm and, in some, pacing rhythms. The wide fixed splitting seen in complete right bundle branch block results from delayed tricuspid closure due to delay in stimulation. In ventricular premature contractions and ventricular tachycardia, the asynchronous contraction of the ventricles results in the wide split S_1. Mechanical delays in mitral or tricuspid closure that may cause wide splitting of S_1 include mitral stenosis, Ebstein's anomaly, and right or left atrial myxomas.

❖   Listen to a wide split S_1 as compared with a normal split S_1 and a single S_1.

EJECTION SOUNDS   S₁ E   S₂

Ejection sounds are high frequency "clicking" sounds that occur very shortly after the S_1. They are usually heard at either base right or base left. These sounds may be of either *aortic* or *pulmonic* origin and are produced when blood is ejected from the right ventricle or left ventricle either through a stenotic valve or into a dilated chamber. Because they are high in frequency, they are heard best with a diaphragm applied firmly.

Pulmonic ejection sounds are heard best at base left but may be heard anywhere along the LLSB (Fig. 9-1, *A*). This sound may increase with expiration and decrease with inspiration in a patient with pulmonary stenosis. The exact reason for this respiratory variation is unknown. It may relate to pressure/volume changes between the right ventricle and pulmonary artery with respiration or be caused by the stenosed pulmonary valve opening with a " snap."

Besides being heard in pulmonic stenosis, the pulmonic ejection sound may also be heard in pulmonary hypertension, atrial septal defects, pulmonary embolism, hyperthyroidism, or in conditions causing enlargement of the pulmonary artery.

❖   Listen now to a pulmonic ejection sound compared to a single S_1.

Fig. 9-1. Area for auscultating ejection sounds (E) and respiratory effect: **A,** *pulmonic ejection sound* (E), which decreases in intensity with inspiration and increases in intensity with expiration; **B,** *aortic ejection sound* (E), which is not effected by respiration. (Modified with permission from L. Caccamo and B. Erickson, *Cardiac Auscultation*, Youngstown, Ohio: St. Elizabeth Hospital Medical Center, 1975.)

Aortic ejection sounds are heard best at the apex but may be heard anywhere on a straight line from base right to the apex. This sound is not affected by respiration. It is heard in valvular aortic stenosis, aortic insufficiency, coarctation of the aorta, and aneurysm of the ascending aorta. (Fig. 9-1, *B*).

❖   Listen now to an aortic ejection sound compared to a single S_1.

MIDSYSTOLIC CLICKS

S_1 C S_2

"Clicks" are high frequency sounds that may be isolated or multiple sounds. Although the click usually occurs in the middle of systole, it may also occur in early or late systole. It occurs at least 0.14 second after S_1.

The most common cause of a midsystolic click or clicks is the ballooning of one of the mitral valve leaflets (usually the posterior one) into the left atrium at the point of maximal ventricular ejection. The click is heard when the chordae tendineae, which may be longer than normal, suddenly stops the ballooning leaflet. This is descriptive of mitral valve prolapse and is the most common cause of the midsystolic click.

Since the clicks are usually of mitral valve origin, they are heard best at the apex. Or they may be heard toward the left sternal border when the posterior leaflet is primarily involved.

❖   Listen now to a midsystolic click compared to a single S_1.

❖   Factors that reduce ventricular volume (standing, valsalva, tachycardia, or amyl nitrite) will cause the click to move closer to S_1. With reduced

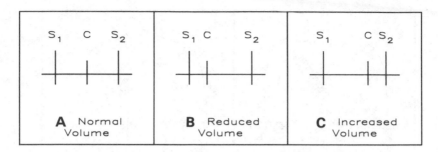

Fig. 9–2. Correlation of click's distance to S₁ and ventricular volume: **A**, *normal* ventricular volume (click in *mid–*systole); **B**, *reduced* ventricular volume (click is *closer* to S₁); **C**, *increased* ventricular volume (click is *farther* from S₁).

ventricular volume, the mitral valve closes earlier after the S_1, and therefore the click moves closer to S_1.

Factors that increase ventricular volume (squatting, bradycardia, propranolol, pressors) will cause the click to move farther from S_1. With increased ventricular volume, mitral valve closure occurs later, and the click, therefore moves further from S_1 (Fig. 9-2).

For a summary of the various sounds that can occur around S_1 and a method of differentiating one from the other, see Table 9-1.

CLINICAL CORRELATION

The stethoscope is still the best instrument to detect and diagnose a prolapse of the mitral valve that occurs in as many as fifteen million Americans. Careful listening is necessary to hear the click and the late systolic murmur (see Chapter 10) that are typically transient, intermittent, and varying. Heart disease in mitral valve prolapse is more frequently absent than present, and the majority of individuals with the syndrome are asymptomatic. Since individuals with mitral valve prolapse have increased risk of developing infective endocarditis following invasive procedures, prophylactic antibiotics are recommended before dental procedures (including cleaning, filling, and extractions), surgical procedures, and invasive procedures of the gastrointestinal and genitourinary tracts.

In the clinical setting, pay particular attention to S_1 and to "sounds around the first sound." Can you differentiate a normal split S_1 from a wide split S_1; from a midsystolic click; from ejection sounds—aortic or pulmonic; from S_4? Use Table 9-1 to help you in your differentiation.

Table 9-1. Differential for sounds around the first heart sound (S₁)

Sound Heard	Area Heard Loudest	Respiratory Variation	Chest Piece*	Change c̄ Pressure on Bell	Listen at Base R	
					S₁ Split?	S₂ Split?
Normal Split	LLSB	↑ Inspiration	D	None	No	Normal
RBBB	LLSB	↑ Inspiration	D	None	No	Wide
S₄ Rt	LLSB	↑ Inspiration	B	Decrease	No	Normal
S₄ Lt	Apex	↓ Inspiration ↑ Expiration	B	Decrease	No	Normal
Ejection Pulmonic	Base L	↓ Inspiration ↑ Expiration	D	None	Yes	Wide
Ejection Aortic	Apex	None	D	None	Yes	Wide

*D = diaphragm chest piece; B = bell chest piece.

(Modified with permission from L. Caccamo and B. Erickson, *Cardiac Auscultation*, Youngstown, Ohio: St. Elizabeth Hospital Medical Center, 1975.)

═══ SELF-LEARNING "UNKNOWN" HEART SOUNDS

❖ On the tape, listen to the "unknown" heart sounds and identify the sound. Compare your answers with the answer key at the end of the chapter. Relisten to the tape as needed to achieve mastery of the content.
You are listening to the heart at base left with the diaphragm, applied firmly:

1. Is S_1 a normal split S_1 or a wide split S_1?

> You are listening to a heart with the diaphragm applied firmly:
> At the LLSB, what do you hear?
> At the apex, what do you hear?
> At base right, what do you hear?
> At base left, what do you hear?

2. The sound you hear around S_1 is a:
   a. normal split S_1 b. wide split S_1
   c. aortic ejection sound   d. pulmonic ejection sound

> You are listening to a heart with the diaphragm firmly pressed:
> At the LLSB, what do you hear?
> At the apex, what do you hear?
> At base right, what do you hear?   ·
> At base left, what do you hear?

3. The sound you hear around S_1 is:
   a. normal split S_1 b. wide split S_1
   c. aortic ejection sound   d. pulmonic ejection sound

> You are listening to a heart with the diaphragm applied firmly:
> At the LLSB, what do you hear?
> At the apex, what do you hear?
> At base right, what do you hear?
> At base left, what do you hear?

4. The sound you hear around S_1 is a:
   a. normal split S_1 b. wide split S_1
   c. aortic ejection sound   d. midsystolic click

> You are listening to the heart at the apex:
> At the LLSB, what do you hear?
> At the apex, what do you hear?
> At base right, what do you hear?
> At base left, what do you hear?

5. The sound you hear around S_1 is a:
   a. normal split S_1 b. aortic ejection sound
   c. S_4 d. midsystolic click

=== **SELF-LEARNING QUESTIONS**

Select the letter of the correct response. Compare your answers with the answer key at the end of the chapter. Reread the chapter as needed to achieve mastery of the content.

1. In right bundle branch block or ventricular tachycardia, which of the following will be heard?
   a. normal split S$_1$
   b. wide split S$_1$
   c. pulmonic ejection sound
   d. midsystolic click

2. A high-frequency sound that occurs very shortly after S$_1$ and is heard anywhere on a straight line from base right to the apex is descriptive of a
   a. wide split S$_1$
   b. midsystolic click
   c. aortic ejection sound
   d. pulmonic ejection sound

3. In a midsystolic click, factors that reduce ventricular volume will cause the click to
   a. disappear
   b. become louder
   c. move further from S$_1$
   d. move closer to S$_1$

4. A wide split S$_1$ is heard best at
   a. base right
   b. base left
   c. apex
   d. left lateral sternal border

5. A midsystolic click is heard best at
   a. base right
   b. base left
   c. apex
   d. left lateral sternal border

=== **ANSWERS TO SELF-LEARNING "UNKNOWN" HEART SOUNDS**

1. Wide split S$_1$

2. c

3. d

4. d

5. c

ANSWERS TO SELF-LEARNING QUESTIONS

1. b

2. c

3. d

4. d

5. c

CHAPTER 10

Sounds Around S_2

LEARNING OBJECTIVES

After reading this chapter, listening to the accompanying tape, answering the self-learning questions at the end of the chapter, and listening to the "unknowns" on the tape, the learner will be able to do the following:

1. Identify the characteristics of a paradoxical split S_2
2. Identify the characteristics of a widely split S_2
3. Identify the characteristics of a fixed split S_2
4. Identify the characteristics of a narrow split S_2
5. Identify the following:
   a. physiological split S_2
   b. paradoxical split S_2
   c. wide split S_2
   d. fixed split S_2
   e. narrow split S_2
   f. S_3
   g. opening snap

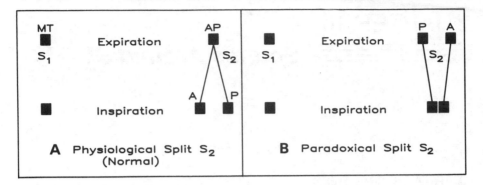

Fig. 10-1. Paradoxical splitting of the second heart sound (S_2): **A**, physiological split S_2, which splits on *inspiration*, is compared to **B**, paradoxical split S_2, which splits on *expiration*. (Reproduced with permission from L. Caccamo and B. Erickson, *Cardiac Auscultation*, Youngstown, Ohio: St. Elizabeth Hospital Medical Center, 1975.)

PARADOXICAL SPLIT S_2

If the closure of the aortic valve is delayed, there may be a reversal of normal closure sequence of S_2, with pulmonic closure (P_2) occurring before aortic closure (A_2) (Fig. 10-1) Paradoxical splitting of S_2 is never heard in the absence of a heart abnormality.

A paradoxical split S_2 is identified clinically when during inspiration there is a single S_2 and during expiration a split S_2. Paradoxical, or reversed, splitting of S_2 may occur with marked volume or pressure loads on the left ventricle (severe aortic stenosis, severe aortic regurgitation, and large patent ductus arteriosus). With the increased volume in the left ventricle, ventricular emptying is delayed, thus delaying closure of the aortic valve. It also occurs in conduction defects that delay left ventricular depolarization (complete left bundle branch block). Conduction defects that delay left ventricular depolarization also delay left ventricular emptying, thus also delaying closure of the aortic valve.

❖   Listen now to a paradoxical split S_2—split audible on expiration; single on inspiration.

WIDE SPLIT S_2

The normal physiological split S_2 can be accentuated by conditions that cause abnormal delay in pulmonic valve closure. Five such conditions are

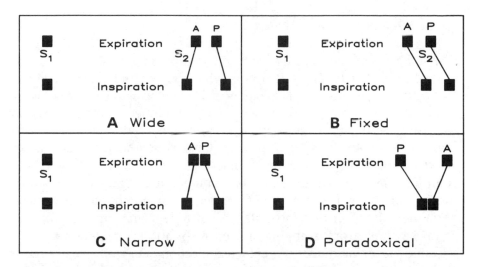

Fig. 10–2. Splitting of the second heart sound (S₂): **A**, wide; **B**, fixed; **C**, narrow; **D**, paradoxical. (Reproduced with permission from L. Caccamo and B. Erickson, *Cardiac Auscultation*, Youngstown, Ohio: St. Elizabeth Hospital Medical Center, 1975.)

1. Increased volume in right ventricle as compared with the left (atrial septal defect, ventricular septal defect).
2. Chronic outflow tract obstruction to the right ventricle (pulmonary stenosis).
3. Acute or chronic dilation of the right ventricle caused by sudden rise in pulmonary artery pressure (pulmonary embolism).
4. Electrical delay or activation of right ventricle (complete right bundle branch block).
5. Decreased elastic recoil of pulmonary artery (idiopathic dilation of the pulmonary artery).

Early closure of the aortic valve may also contribute to a widely split S₂. Mitral insufficiency may cause early closure of the aortic valve, since some of the left ventricular output is regurgitated into the atrium.

The wide split has a duration of 0.04 to 0.05 second. The physiological (normal) split is 0.03 second (Fig. 10-2, A).

❖   Listen now to a wide split S₂. Compare it to a normal split S₂ and a single S₂.

FIXED SPLIT S₂

A split that does not change its width with inspiration or expiration is called a fixed split (Fig.10-2, *B*). It occurs when the ventricles are unable to change their volumes with respiration. This can occur in congestive heart failure, cardiomyopathy, atrial septal defect, or ventricular septal defect. In congestive heart failure the congested lungs cannot withhold much blood from the left ventricle during inspiration; thus left ventricular volume is not markedly affected by respiration. Another factor is that a dilated and poorly compliant left ventricle, which is common to congestive failure or cardiomyopathy, may not be able to respond to small changes in volume. Atrial septal defect or ventricular septal defect may prevent the left ventricle alone from changing size on respiration. Or there may be a selective shortening of the left ventricular ejection time with an early aortic closure, as in severe mitral insufficiency or ventricular septal defect.

❖   Listen now to a fixed split S₂. Compare it to a physiological split S₂.

NARROW SPLIT S₂

A narrow split S₂ may be heard in conditions that cause increased left ventricular volume without markedly affecting the right side (uncomplicated patent ductus arteriosus with aortic regurgitation). It may also be heard in conditions causing obstruction to outflow of the left ventricle (aortic stenosis or electrical delay, as in left bundle branch block). The above conditions would cause delay in the closure of the aortic valve but would not delay closure of the pulmonic valve (A₂ closer to P₂).

     With aging, the pulmonary component comes earlier, and the split narrows. This occurs because there is less blood pooling in the lungs (A₂ closer to P₂) and less venous return (P₂ closer to A₂) (Fig. 10-2, *C*).

❖   Listen to narrow split S₂. Compare it to a physiological split S₂.

OPENING SNAP

Normally the opening of the mitral valve is not discernible, but under certain conditions the opening is audible and becomes known as the opening snap—a short, high-frequency click or snap that occurs after the second S₂. It is the result of an audible opening of the mitral valve due to stiffening (mitral stenosis) or increased flow (ventricular septal defect or patent ductus arteriosus). It is best heard between the apex and the LLSB with the diaphragm applied firmly. During inspiration the opening snap is softer (because of decreased blood return to the left ventricle.) With increased tricuspid flow, as in atrial septal defect, a tricuspid opening snap may be heard. It is a high-frequency sound heard loudest at LLSB with the diaphragm applied firmly. The tricuspid opening snap becomes louder with inspiration.

The opening snap is one of the early signs of mitral stenosis, and initially the opening snap is widely separated from S_2 (making it easy to hear). As the left atrial pressure increases, the opening to the mitral valve occurs earlier in diastole; therefore the opening snap moves closer to S_2. (You may then confuse it with a split S_2. But opening snap is higher frequency and more "clicky" than S_2). In very severe stenosis the opening snap may merge with the components of S_2.

❖   Listen now to an S_2 followed by an opening snap.

DIFFERENTIATING S_3 FROM THE OPENING SNAP

❖ The opening snap occurs earlier after S_2 and is a **high**-frequency sound best heard with the diaphragm applied firmly. S_3 occurs later than the opening snap, following S_2 and is a **low**-frequency sound best heard with the bell held lightly. For a synopsis of the various sounds that can occur around the S_2 and a method of differentiating one from the other, see Table 10-1.

CLINICAL CORRELATION

In the clinical setting, pay particular attention to S_2 and the "sounds around the second." Can you differentiate a physiological split S_2 from a paradoxical split S_2; from a wide split S_2; from a fixed split S_2; from a narrow split S_2; from S_3; from an opening snap? Use Table 10-1 to help you in your differentiation.

A technique taught by Harvey can be used to develop and sharpen your ability to detect degrees of splitting. Use your knuckles or fingers and strike two knuckles or fingers against a hard surface. By varying the degree of asynchrony, you can accurately simulate degrees of splitting from close to wide. If you use only one knuckle or finger, a single sound is simulated. (This same technique can be used to simulate S_1, S_2, S_3, S_4, or an opening snap.)

Table 10-1. Differential for sounds around the second heart sound (S_2)

Sound Heard	Area Heard Loudest	Respiratory Variation	Chest Piece*	Change $\bar{c}$ Pressure on Bell
normal split	Base L	Heard on inspiration	D	No
wide split	Base L	Heard on inspiration	D	No
fixed split	Base L	None	D	No
narrow split	Base L	Heard on inspiration	D	No
paradoxical split	Base L	Heard on expiration	D	No
opening snap	Apex or LLSB	↓ inspiration ↑ expiration	D	No
S_3Rt	Xiphoid or LLSB	↑ inspiration	B	Yes
S_3Lt	Apex	↓ inspiration ↑ expiration	B	Yes

*D = diaphragm chest piece; B = bell chest piece.

(Modified with permission from L. Caccamo and B. Erickson, *Cardiac Ausculta-tion,* Youngstown, Ohio: St. Elizabeth Hospital Medical Center, 1975.)

═══ **SELF-LEARNING "UNKNOWN" HEART SOUNDS**

❖ On the tape, listen to the "unknown" heart sounds and identify the sound. Compare your answers with the answer key at the end of the chapter. Relisten to the tape as needed to achieve mastery of the content.

You are listening to the heart at base left with the diaphragm applied firmly:

1. Is the S_2 splitting physiologically or paradoxically?

2. Is the S_2 splitting physiologically or paradoxically?

3. Is S_2 wide or narrow?

    You are listening to the heart at the apex:
        Using the bell held lightly, what do you hear?
        Using the bell applied firmly, what do you hear?
        Using the diaphragm applied firmly, what do you hear?
4. Is there an S_3 or a widely split S_2?

You are listening to the heart at the apex:
    Using the bell held lightly, what do you hear?
    Using the bell applied firmly, what do you hear?
    Using the diaphragm applied firmly, what do you hear?
5. Is there an S_3 or an opening snap?

SELF-LEARNING QUESTIONS

Select the letter of the correct response. Compare your answers with the answer
key at the end of the chapter. Reread the chapter as needed to achieve mastery of
the content.

1. The reversal of the normal closure sequence of S_2 with the pulmonic closure
   (P_2) occurring before aortic closure (A_2) is descriptive of a
   a. physiologically split S_2 **b.** paradoxically split S_2
   c. widely split S_2 **d.** narrowly split S_2

2. Abnormal delay in pulmonic valve closure (P_2) is descriptive of a
   a. physiologically split S_2 **b.** paradoxically split S_2
   c. widely split S_2 **d.** narrowly split S_2

3. A split of S_2 that does not change its width with inspiration or expiration is
   descriptive of a
   a. physiologically split S_2 **b.** paradoxically split S_2
   c. fixed split S_2 **d.** narrowly split S_2

4. A split of S_2 in which the pulmonic component (P_2) comes earlier than normal
   is descriptive of a
   a. physiologically split S_2 **b.** paradoxically split S_2
   c. fixed split S_2 **d.** narrowly split S_2

5. A short, high-frequency sound that occurs after S_2 and is the result of the
   audible opening of the mitral valve as a result of stiffness is descriptive of a(n)
   a. physiologically split S_2 **b.** paradoxically split S_2
   c. fixed split S_2 **d.** opening snap after S_2

ANSWERS TO SELF-LEARNING "UNKNOWN" HEART SOUNDS

  1. Physiologically split S_2

  2. Paradoxically split S_2

3. Wide split S_2

4. S_3

5. Opening snap

ANSWERS TO SELF-LEARNING QUESTIONS

1. b

2. c

3. c

4. b

5. d

CHAPTER 11

Friction Rubs— Pericardial and Pleural

LEARNING OBJECTIVES

After reading this chapter, listening to the accompanying tape, answering the self-learning questions at the end of the chapter, and listening to the "unknowns" on the tape, the learner will be able to do the following:

1. Identify the common etiologies of a pericardial friction rub
2. Identify the auscultatory signs of a pericardial friction rub
3. Identify the sound characteristics of a pericardial friction rub
4. Identify the common etiologies of a pleural friction rub
5. Identify the auscultatory signs of a pleural friction rub
6. Identify the sound characteristics of a pleural friction rub
7. Differentiate a pericardial friction rub from a pleural friction rub

To differentiate between pericardial and pleural friction rubs, the listener must consider the following factors.

PERICARDIAL FRICTION RUBS

Etiologies

A pericardial friction rub is a sign of pericardial inflammation. Some common etiologies include the following:

1. **Infective pericarditis.** Many organisms may cause infective pericariditis. Common ones include viral, pyogenic, tubercular, and myocotic.
2. **Noninfective pericarditis.** Myocardial infarction, uremia, neoplasms, myxedema, open heart surgery, and trauma are some of the non-infective causes of a pericardial friction rub.
3. **Autoimmune problems.** Rheumatic fever, collagen vascular disease, drug-induced (i.e. procainamide) injury, and postmyocardial injury (Dressler's syndrome) are autoimmune causes of pericardial friction.

Auscultatory Signs

The auscultatory signs of a pericardial friction rub are **one systolic sound** and **two diastolic sounds.** The **systolic** sound (between S_1 and S_2) may occur anywhere in systole. The two **diastolic** sounds occur at the times the ventricles are stretched in diastole:

1. In early diastole near the end of the early diastolic filling. (This is the same time that an S_3 would occur.)
2. At end diastole, when atrial contraction produces sudden ventricular expansion. (This is the same time that an S_4 would occur.) If atrial contraction does not occur, as in atrial fibrillation, the second diastolic sound is *not* heard.

Sound Characteristics

1. The pericardial friction rub has a scratching, grating, or squeaking, to-and-fro leathery quality.
2. This rub is *high* in frequency and therefore heard best with the *diaphragm* chestpiece applied firmly.

3. The pericardial friction rub tends to be louder during **inspiration.** This may be due to the following:
   a. The downward pull of the diaphragm on the pericardium during inspiration, which causes the pericardium to be drawn more tautly over the heart during inspiration
   b. The expanded lung pressing on the pericardium
   c. The fact that the pericardium is stretched more during inspiration than during expiration because the expansion of the right ventricle is greater during inspiration than that of the left ventricle during expiration
4. The pericardial friction rub may be most audible in some patients during **forced expiration** with the patient leaning forward or on hands and knees. (These manuevers cause less air to be between the pericardium and the stethoscope and also bring the heart closer to the chest wall.)
5. The pericardial friction rub is likely to be transitory or inconstant. This means that it comes and goes suddenly.
6. The pericardial rub may be heard anywhere on the pericardium but it is often loudest at the LLSB.
7. Most patients with a pericardial friction rub also have a tachycardia.

❖   Listen to a pericardial friction rub with a heart rate of 60 beats per minute with both systolic and diastolic sounds.

❖   Listen to a heart rate of 60 beats per minute. Then only the systolic component of the rub will be added.

❖   Listen to a heart rate of 60 beats per minute. Then only the diastolic components of the rub will be added.

❖   Now listen to a heart rate 60 beats per minute. First the systolic component of the rub will be added and then the diastolic components.

❖   Now listen to a pericardial friction rub at a heart rate of 120 beats per minute.

❖   Listen to a real heart with a pericardial friction rub; all three components are present.

PLEURAL FRICTION RUBS

Etiologies

A pleural friction rub is a sign of pleural inflammation and indicates that the visceral and parietal surfaces of the pleura are rubbing together. Some common etiologies causing pleural friction rubs are:

1. Pneumonia
2. Viral Infections
3. Tuberculosis
4. Pulmonary Embolism

Auscultatory Signs

The auscultatory signs of a pleural friction rub are **one sound during inspiration** and **one sound during expiration** (this may not always be heard).

Sound Characteristics

1. The pleural friction rub has a grating or creaking sound similar to that heard in the pericardical friction rub.
2. This rub is *high* in frequency and therefore is best heard with the *diaphragm* chestpiece applied firmly.
3. The pleural friction rub is heard during inspiration and sometimes during expiration. (The expiratory component may be absent.)
4. The pleural friction rub commonly is heard in the lower anterolateral chest wall (the area of greatest thoracic mobility) on the side of the pleural inflammation.
5. The pleural friction rub decreases with a decrease in lung movement. The sound disappears if the breath is held.
6. The pleural friction rub has a superficial character. It sounds closer to the surface than does a pericardial friction rub.

❖   Listen to a pleural friction rub from a real individual. Note the inspiratory and expiratory components.

❖   Compare the pleural friction rub to a pericardial friction rub. First a pleural friction rub, then a pericardial friction rub.

**SUMMARY FOR DIFFERENTIATING PERICARDIAL AND PLEURAL
FRICTION RUBS**

	Pericardial	**Pleural**
Frequency	High	High
Quality	Scratching, grating, squeaking	Grating or creaking
Chestpiece best heard with	Diaphragm	Diaphragm
Timing	One sytolic sound; two diastolic sounds	One sound inspiration one sound expiration (this may be absent)
	Transitory	Transitory (but less abrupt)
Site	Over pericardium (left chest)	Over anterolateral chest—right or left side
Respiratory variant	Louder during inspiration	Decrease with decrease in breathing; gone when breath held
Surface proximity	Further from surface	Superficial; closer to surface

CLINICAL CORRELATION

In the clinical setting seek out patients with pericardial friction rubs and pleural friction rubs. Use the above chart to help you in your differentiation. Compare the sounds of the friction rubs with those of systolic and diastolic murmurs. Practice charting your findings. If you have difficulty in differentiating pericardial friction rubs from pleural friction rubs, ask the patient to stop breathing. (It is a good idea to hold your own breath at the same time so that you remember to permit the patient to again breath.) If during respiratory cessation the sound goes away, it is a pleural rub; if the sound remains, it is a pericardial rub.

≡≡≡   **SELF-LEARNING "UNKNOWN" HEART SOUNDS**

❖   On the tape, listen to the "unknown" heart sounds and identify the sound. Compare your answers with the answer key at the end of the chapter. Relisten to the tape as needed to achieve mastery of the content.

You are listening at the LLSB. You hear the following sound.

1. You identify the sound as a
    a. pericardial friction rub   **b.** pleural friction rub
    c. systolic murmur   **d.** diastolic murmur

You are listening at the apex. You hear the following sound.
2. You identify the sound as a
    a. pericardial friction rub   **b.** pleural friction rub
    c. systolic murmur   **d.** diastolic murmur

≡≡≡   **SELF-LEARNING QUESTIONS**

Select the letter of the correct response. Compare your answers with the answer key at the end of the chapter. Reread the chapter as needed to achieve mastery of the content.

1. Identify two of the common etiologies of a pericardial friction rub.
    a.
    b.

2. One of the diastolic sounds of the pericardial friction rub occurs in early diastole; the other occurs at
    a. mid-diastole   **b.** late diastole
    c. rapid diastolic filling   **d.** none of the above

3. Identify two of the common etiologies of a pleural friction rub in early diastole.
    a.
    b.

4. Which characteristic is most helpful in differentiating a pericardial from a pleural friction rub?
    a. quality   **b.** frequency
    c. breath-holding   **d.** site

ANSWERS TO SELF-LEARNING "UNKNOWN" HEART SOUNDS

1. a

2. b

ANSWERS TO SELF-LEARNING QUESTIONS

1. Any two of the following:
    —Infective (e.g., viral, tuberculosis)
    —Noninfective (e.g., myocardial infarction)
    —Autoimmune (rheumatic fever)

2. b

3. Any two of the following:
    —Pneumonia
    —Viral infections
    —Tuberculosis
    —Pulmonary embolism

4. c

Bibliography

Alspach JG (ed): *Core curriculum for critical care nursing,* ed 4, Philadelphia, 1990, WB Saunders.

Caccamo L, Erickson B: *Cardiac auscultation,* Youngstown, Ohio, 1975, St. Elizabeth Hospital Medical Center.

Constant J: *Bedside cardiology,* Boston, 1969, Little, Brown.

Erickson B: Detecting abnormal heart sounds, *Nurs 86,* 16(1):58-63, January 1986.

Harris A, et al (eds): *Physiological and clinical aspects of cardiac auscultation,* Philadelphia, 1976, JB Lippincott.

Harvey WP, Canfield DC: *Clinical auscultation of the cardiovascular system: tapes with companion tests,* Newton, NJ, 1989, Laennec Publishing.

Miracle VA: Anatomy of a murmur, *Nurs 86,* 16(7):26-32, July 1986.

Patridge SA: Cardiac auscultation, *Dimensions Crit Care Nurs,* 2(3):152-156, May-June 1982.

Spence JI, Lemberg L: Cardiac auscultation in acute myocardial infarction, *Heart lung,* 10(5):901-905, 1981.

Taylor DL: Assessing heart sounds, *Nurs 85,* 15(1):51-53, January, 1985.

Glossary

A₂: Aortic component of the second heart sound; normally comes before the pulmonic component (P_2).

Aortic ejection sound: *See* Ejection sound, aortic.

Aortic valve: Semilunar valve that prevents the backflow of blood from the aorta into the left ventricle during ventricular diastole. The closure of this valve is responsible for the first component (A_2) of the second heart sound.

Apex: Area of cardiac auscultation. Also known as the point of maximum impulse (PMI) of the heart against the chest wall. In the normal adult it is at the fifth intercostal space to the left of the sternum at the midclavicular line. Sounds from the mitral valve and the left heart are best heard in this area.

Atrial kick: Slang term for atrial systole or atrial contraction that may contibute 20% to 25% to ventricular filling. It occurs during the late filling phase of the ventricular diastolic period but only if atrial contraction occurs. It can never occur in the presence of atrial fibrillation.

Atrial systole: *See* Systole, atrial.

Auscultogram: A graphic method of charting heart sounds.

Base left: Area of cardiac auscultation; the second intercostal space to the left of the sternum. Sounds from the pulmonic valve are best heard in this area.

Base right: Area of cardiac auscultation; the second intercostal space to the right of the sternum. Sounds from the aortic valve are best heard in this area.

Bell chestpiece: Component of the stethoscope that has a shallow shell with a diameter as large as feasible to permit an air seal when held lightly on the chest wall so that no after-imprint is left. It transmits sounds of **low** frequency.

Cardiac cycle: The period from the beginning of one beat of the heart to the beginning of the next succeeding beat; consists of two phases: one of contraction, systole—atrial and ventricular; and one of relaxation, diastole—atrial and ventricular.

Click: High-frequency sound that is heard after the first heart sound (S_1). It may be a single or multiple sound heard in the middle of ventricular systolic period; often associated with mitral valve prolapse.

Compliance: Term meaning the ratio of change in volume to a change in pressure (V/ P). Ventricular compliance is decreased in the presence of any condition that limits the ability of the ventricle(s) to expand. Decreased ventricular compliance is one mechanism responsible for the production of the third (S_3) and the fourth (S_4) heart sounds.

Diaphragm chestpiece: A component of the stethoscope that has a taut (stiff) material drawn across its diameter. When it is firmly applied to the chest wall [leaving an after-imprint], it transmits sounds of high frequency.

Diastolic murmurs: *See* Murmurs, diastolic.

Diastole, ventricular: Period of ventricular filling that follows closure of the aortic and pulmonic valves. The ventricular diastolic period is divided into three phases:

1. The first third of the diastolic period, which has two sub-divisions—the isovolumic relaxation phase and the rapid filling phase
2. The middle third of the diastolic period during which both atrium and ventricles are relaxed
3. The last third of diastole, or the late filling phase, during which atrial contraction takes place.

Duration: The length of time that a sound lasts. Normal heart sounds [S_1 and S_2] are of short duration. Cardiac murmurs or rubs are of long duration.

Ejection murmur: *See* Murmur—mid.

Ejection sound: These are high-frequency "clicking" sounds occurring very shortly after the first sound. They may be of either aortic or pulmonic origin.

Aortic: High-frequency "clicking" sound heard best at the apex but may be heard anywhere on a straight line from base right to the apex. Heard in valvular aortic stenosis, aortic insufficiency, coarctation of the aorta, and aneurysm of the ascending aorta.

Pulmonic: High-frequency "clicking" sound heard best at base left but may be heard anywhere along the left sternal border. It may be heard in pulmonic stenosis, pulmonary hypertension, atrial septal defects, pulmonary embolism, hyperthyroidism, or in conditions causing enlargement of the pulmonary artery.

First heart sound: The initial sound heard—also known as S_1. It occurs at the beginning of ventricular systole when ventricular volume is maximal. It is due to the closure of the mitral (M_1) and tricuspid (T_1)

valves.

Split, normal: When both mitral (M_1) and tricuspid (T_1) closure are distinguishable and are 0.02 second apart.

Split, wide: Mitral and tricuspid closure sounds occur wider apart from either electrical or mechanical causes that result in ventricular asynchrony.

Fourth heart sound: The fourth heart sound is a low-frequency sound heard just before the first heart sound. It is a result of decreased ventricular compliance or increased volume of filling. It is also known as an "atrial gallop," "presystolic gallop," "S_4 gallop," or "S_4."

Frequency: The number of wave cycles generated per second by a vibrating body. It is the vibratory movement of an object in motion that initiates the sound wave cycles that can be discerned by the stethoscope.

Frequency, high: The greater the number of wave cycles per second generated by a vibrating body, the higher is the frequency. Sounds of high frequency are best heard with the diaphragm chestpiece firmly pressed.

Frequency, low: The fewer the number of wave cycles per second generated by a vibrating body, the lower the frequency. Sounds of low frequency are best heard with the bell lightly applied.

Frequency, mid: Combination of high and low frequencies. Sound heard equally well with either bell or diaphragm.

Heart sound simulator: An electronic device designed to generate all normal and abnormal heart sound patterns by the independent variation of all sound parameters.

Intensity: Is related to the height of the sound wave produced by a vibrating object. Intensity determines the loudness of the perceived sound. Objects vibrating with great energy are heard as loud sounds. Objects vibrating with low energy are heard as soft sounds.

Isovolumic contaction: A phase during the first part of ventricular systole. It begins with the first initial rise in ventricular pressure after the closure of the mitral and tricuspid valves.

Isovolumic relaxation: A phase during the first third of the ventricular diastole. Intially in this period no blood is entering the ventricles, and the ventricles therefore are not increasing in volume.

Late filling phase: Phase during the last third of ventricular diastole. It is at this time that the "atrial kick" or atrial contraction takes place.

Left lateral recumbent: Position for cardiac auscultation in which patient is lying on his/her left side with left arm extended under head. The heart is brought closer to the chest wall in this position. Also the exertion of turning to this position increases heart rate. This position may be useful in making audible the diastolic rumble of mitral stenosis, the low-frequency third heart sound (S_3), of congestive heart failure.

Left lateral sternal border: Area of cardiac auscultation which is at the left fifth intercostal space in the mid-clavicular line. Sounds from the tricuspid valve and right heart are best heard in this area.

M_1: The mitral component of the first heart sound. This is normally the first component and occurs just after the mitral valve closes; normally comes before the tricuspid component (T_1).

Mitral valve: Bicuspid valve between the left atrium and the left ventricle; one of two "A-V valves"; prevents backflow of blood from left ventricle to left atrium during ventricular systole. Closure of this valve is responsible for the first component (M_1) of the first heart sound.

Mitral valve prolapse: Syndrome associated with a mid-systolic click and a late systolic murmur. One of the mitral leaflets, usually the posterior one, balloons into the left atrium at the point of maximal ventricular ejection. The click is heard when the chordae tendinae suddenly stops the ballooning leaflet. If the leaflets pull apart, a late systolic murmur of mitral regurgitation may also be heard. Also known as "Barlow's syndrome," "floppy mitral valve," or "click-murmur syndrome."

Murmurs: Sustained noises that are audible during the time periods of systole, diastole, or both.

> **Diastolic murmur:** Sustained noises that are audible between the second heart sound (S_2) and the next first heart sound (S_1). They should be considered organic and not normal. Common causes include mitral or tricuspid stenosis and aortic or pulmonic regurgitation.

> **Early:** Peaks in the first third of the cycle.

> **Mid:** Peaks in the middle of the cycle; crescendo-decrescendo ("diamond shaped"). Also known as "ejection" murmur.

> **Late:** Peaks in the later third of the cycle.

> **Pan:** Heard continuously throughout the cycle.

> **Systolic murmur:** Sustained noises that are audible between the first (S_1) and the second (S_2) heart sounds. Common causes include mitral or tricuspid regurgitation and aortic or pulmonic stenosis.

Opening snap: Short, high frequency click or "snap" that occurs after the second heart sound. It is most often produced by the opening of a stenosed, thickened, or distorted mitral or tricuspid valve.

P_2: Pulmonic component of the second heart sound (S_2); usually follows aortic component (A_2).

Pitch: Subjective sensation that indicates to the listener whether the tone is high or low on a musical scale.

Point of maximal impulse: Area on the chest at which the heart is best palpable; usually corresponds to apex, which in a normal adult is located at the fifth intercostal space, midclavicular line, to the left of the sternum.

Pulmonic ejection sound: *See* Ejection sound, pulmonic.

Pulmonic valve: Semilunar valve that prevents backflow of blood from the pulmonary artery into the right ventricle during ventricular diastole. Closure of the valve is responsible for the second component (P_2) of the second heart sound.

Quality: This is a sound characteristic that distinguishes two sounds that have equal degrees of frequency and intensity but come from a different source—e.g., piano from a violin, or heart from lung.

   Blow: Mainly high frequency.

   Harsh: Mix of high and low frequencies—slightly more high than low.

   Rough: Mix of high and low frequencies—slightly more low than high.

   Rumble: Mainly low frequency.

Rapid filling phase: Phase during the first third of ventricular diastole. It occurs when ventricular pressure is less than atrial pressure. The mitral and tricuspid valves then open, and blood rapidly enters the ventricles.

Rapid ventricular ejection: Phase during the first part of ventricular systole. It follows the isovolumic contraction phase. It occurs when ventricular pressure exceeds the pressure in the aorta and the pulmonary artery and forces the aortic and pulmonic valves open and blood is rapidly ejected from the ventricles.

S_1: *See* First heart sound.

S_2: *See* Second heart sound.

S_3: *See* Third heart sound.

S_4: *See* Fourth heart sound.

Second heart sound: Second sound heard in a normal heart— also known as S_2. It occurs at the end of ventricular systole. It is due to the closure of the aortic (A_2) and pulmonic (P_2) valves.

   Split, fixed: This split does not change its width with inspiration or expiration.

   Split, narrow: The aortic (A_2) and pulmonic (P_2) components are closer together than normal—<0.03 second. The split is heard on **inspiration** and is single on expiration.

   Split, physiological: The aortic (A_2) and pulmonic (P_2) components that make up the second sound are separately distinguishable— 0.03 second apart. The split is heard on **inspiration** and is single on expiration.

   Split, paradoxical: Reversal of the normal closure sequence of S_2, with pulmonic closure (P_2) occurring before aortic closure (A_2). This split is heard during **expiration** and becomes single on inspiration. (The opposite of a normal or physiological split.)

   Split, wide: Delay in pulmonic valve closure can cause the physiological split to be accentuated or increased—0.04 to 0.05 second. The split is heard during **inspiration** and becomes single on expiration.

Sine wave: An up and down or to and fro undulating or wavy line.

Split: When both components that make up a sound are separately distinguishable, the sound is said to "split." A duration of 0.02 second between the sounds is necessary for the ear to be able to make this distinction. See first sound, split and/or second sound, split.

Stethoscope: Acoustical instrument that uses the vibration of sounds reacting on the air column enclosed in tubing to transmit sounds to the listener's ear. When used for heart sounds, a bell and diaphragm chestpiece are necessary.

Systole, atrial: Period in cardiac cycle. It occurs during the last third of ventricular diastole or during the late filling phase. During this period contraction of the atrium takes place, and the remaining blood is squeezed from the atrium. This is also known as the "atrial kick." Atrial systole may contribute 20% to 25% to ventricular filling. The contribution is less at faster heart rates—100 beats per minute or greater.

Systole, ventricular: Period in cardiac cycle. It follows closure of the mitral and tricuspid valves. This systolic period is divided into two phases: (1) The first phase includes the isovolumic contraction phase and the rapid ventricular ejection phase. (2) During the latter part of ventricular systole, ventricular pressure falls, and reduced ventricular ejection occurs. This period lasts until ventricular ejection stops and ventricular diastole begins.

Systolic murmurs: *See* Murmurs, systolic.

T_1: Second component of the first sound. It normally occurs after M_1 (the mitral component) just after the tricuspid valve closes.

Third heart sound: Low-frequency sound heard just after the second heart sound. It is a diastolic sound that occurs during the early rapid filling phase of ventricular diastole. It is a result of decreased ventricular compliance or increased ventricular diastolic volume. It is also known as a "ventricular gallop," "protodiastolic gallop," "S_3 gallop," or "S_3."

Thrill: Continuous palpable sensation felt on the precordium. It is comparable to the vibration felt when a cat purrs.

Thrust: Palpable (sometimes even visible) intermittent sensation. This is the sensation felt when palpating the point of maximal impulse (PMI) at the apex of the heart.

Timing: Determining whether sound is occurring during systolic or diastolic period.

Timing, finer: Determining whether sound is occurring early, mid, or late in the systolic or diastolic period.

Tricuspid valve: Three-leaflet valve between the right atrium and the right ventricle: one of two "A-V" valves; prevents backflow of blood from the right ventricle to right atrium during ventricular systole. Closure of this valve is responsible for the second component (T_1) of the first heart sound.

Turbulence: Smooth blood flow is disturbed, and the blood flows crosswise in the vessel or chamber, as well as along the vessel. This causes eddy currents similar to a whirlpool and produces vibrations that are audible.

Ventricular diastole: *See* Diastole, ventricular.

Ventricular systole: *See* Systole, ventricular.

Index

A

A_1, intensity of, 21
A_2
  intensity of, 30, 31
  in paradoxical split S_2, 78
Acceleration of blood, heart sounds and,
    8
Amplifying stethoscopes, 11
Amplitude of sound, 10
Amyl nitrate, inhalation of, murmurs and,
    52
Anemia
  innocent systolic murmurs in, 57
  and S_4, 36
Aneurysm of ascending aorta, aortic
    ejection sounds in, 71
Aorta
  ascending, aneurysm of, aortic ejection
    sounds in, 71
  coarctation of, aortic ejection sounds
    in, 71
Aortic area of heart, auscultation at, 5
Aortic ejection sounds, 71, 73
Aortic insufficiency, aortic ejection
    sounds in, 71
Aortic regurgitation
  diastolic murmurs caused by, 64, 66
  differentiation of, by pitch and quality,
    51
  murmur of, 51
    maneuvers to differentiate, 52
  narrow split S_2 in, 80
  paradoxical split S_2 in, 78
Aortic septal defect, differentiation of, by
    pitch and quality, 51
Aortic valve
  incompetence of, diastolic murmurs
    caused by, 64

Aortic valve—cont'd
  murmur at, locating, 48, 49
  stenosis of
    differentiation of, by pitch and
      quality, 49
    mid-systolic murmur in, 57
    murmur of, 51
      maneuvers to differentiate, 52
    narrow split S_2 in, 80
    paradoxical split S_2 in, 78
    and S_4, 36
    systolic murmurs in, 56, 58
    valvular, aortic ejection sounds in,
      71
Aortic valve sounds, 8
Apex of heart, auscultation at, 5
Arteriovenous connection causing
    murmurs, 48
Artery
  coronary, disease of
    S_3 and, 42
    S_4 and, 36
  pulmonary
    enlargement of, pulmonic ejection
      sounds in, 70
    idiopathic dilation of, wide split S_2
      in, 79
Ascending aorta, aneurysm of, aortic
    ejection sounds in, 71
Atrial fibrillation and S_4, 36, 37
Atrial gallop, 36; *see also* Fourth heart
    sound
Atrial myxomas causing wide split S_1, 70
Atrial septal defect
  fixed split S_2 in, 80
  opening snap with, 81
  pulmonic ejection sounds in, 70
  wide split S_2 in, 79
Atrial systole, 7

Atrioventricular block and S_4, 37
Atrioventricular communication, systolic
    murmur with, 56
Atrioventricular shunt causing murmurs,
    48
Auscultation
  basic positions for, 3
  of cardiac valves, sites of, 8
  for high-frequency sounds, 4
  history of, 2
  for low-frequency sounds, 4
  requirements for, 2-6
  of S_2, sites for, 31
  selective listening during, 6
  sequence for, 6
  sites for, 5
  stethoscope for, 4-5
Auscultatory signs of friction rub
  pericardial, 86
  pleural, 88
Auscultogram, 13, 14
Autoimmune problems causing
    pericardial friction rubs, 86

B

Backward regurgitation causing murmurs,
  48
Base of heart, auscultation at, 5
"be" sound, 15
Beats, premature, ventricular, causing
    wide split S_1, 70
Block, atrioventricular, and S_4, 37
Blood, acceleration or deceleration of,
    heart sounds and, 8
Blood flow, turbulent
  factors producing, 9
  heart sounds and, 8-9
"Blowing" murmurs, 50
"bub" sound, 15
Bundle branch block
  left
    narrow split S_2 in, 80
    paradoxical split S_2 in, 78
  right
    causing wide split S_1, 70, 73
    wide split S_2 in, 79
"bup" sound, 15
"bupp" sound, 15

C

Cadence, four-sound, 43
Cardiac cycle, 6, 7
  and heart sounds, relationship between,
    8
Cardiac output, increased, and S_4, 36
Cardiomyopathy
  fixed split S_2 in, 80
  S_3 and, 42
  S_4 and, 36
Cardiovascular physical examination, 2
Carotid pulse and timing of first heart
    sound, 25
Chest, anatomy of, and intensity of S_1, 22,
    23
Children
  innocent systolic murmur in, 56
  S_3 in, 42
  split S_1 in, 21
  systolic murmurs in, 56
Chordae tendineae causing murmurs, 48
Clicks
  definition of, 71
  mid-systolic, 71-72
Coarctation of aorta, aortic ejection
    sounds in, 71
Collagen vascular disease causing
    pericardial friction rubs, 86
Congestive heart failure
  fixed split S_2 in, 80
  S_3 and, 42, 43
Contraction, ventricular, and intensity of
    S_1, 22, 23
Contraction phase, isovolumic, of
    ventricular systole, 7
Coronary artery disease
  S_3 and, 42
  S_4 and, 36
Crescendo murmur, 51
Crescendo/decrescendo murmur, 51

D

"de" sound, 15
Deceleration of blood, heart sounds and,
  8
Decrescendo murmur, 51
Decrescendo/crescendo murmur, 51
Diastole, 7

Diastole,—cont'd
  ventricular, 7
Diastolic murmur(s), 50, 63-68
  definition of, 64
  early, 64
  late, 65
  mechanism of production of, 64
  mid-, 64
  pan-, 65
Diastolic sounds in pericardial friction
      rubs, 86
Diastolic volume, left ventricular,
      increased, S_3 and, 42
Dilation of pulmonary artery, idiopathic,
      wide split S_2 in, 79
Disease
  collagen vascular, causing pericardial
      friction rubs, 86
  coronary artery
    S_3 and, 42
    S_4 and, 36
  heart
    primary, and S_4, 36
    S_3 and, 42
Dressler's syndrome causing pericardial
      friction rubs, 86
Drug-induced injury causing pericardial
      friction rubs, 86
"dub" sound, 15
Ductus arteriosus, patent, 65
  narrow split S_2 in, 80
  opening snap with, 80
  paradoxical split S_2 in, 78
  S_3 and, 42
"dup" sound, 15
"dupp" sound, 15
Duration of sound, 10
Dysrhythmias and S_4, 37

E

Ear, human, and sound transmission, 11-
    12
Early diastolic murmurs, 64
Early innocent systolic murmur, 56
Early murmur, 50
Early systolic murmurs, 56-57
Ebstein's anomaly causing wide split S_1,
    70
Ejection, ventricular, rapid, in ventricular
    systole, 7

Ejection innocent systolic murmur, 56
Ejection murmur, mid-systolic murmur
    as, 57
Ejection sounds, 70-71
  aortic, 71, 73
  pulmonic, 70, 71, 73
Elderly, innocent systolic murmurs in, 57
Embolism, pulmonary
  causing pleural friction rubs, 88
  pulmonic ejection sounds in, 70
  wide split S_2 in, 79
Erb's point, 48, 49
Examination, physical, cardiovascular, 2
Exercise
  innocent systolic murmurs with, 57
  murmurs and, 52
Expiration
  murmurs and, 52
  pericardial friction rubs in, 87
  pleural friction rubs in, 88

F

Fever
  innocent systolic murmurs in, 57
  rheumatic, causing pericardial friction
      rubs, 86
Fibrillation, atrial, and S_4, 36, 37
Filling phase
  late, of ventricular diastole, 7
  rapid, of ventricular diastole, 7
First heart sound, 8, 19-27
  components of, 20
  differentiating, from second heart
      sound, 24-25
  differentiating S_4 from, 73
  intensity of, 21-23
  normal, 22, 32
  sounds around, 69-75
    differentiation of, 73
  split, 20-21
    characteristics of, 37
    differentiating, from S_4, 37
  theories on production of, 20
  wide split, 70
Fixed split S_2, 79, 80, 82
Four-sound cadence, 43
Fourth heart sound, 35-40
  causes of, 36
  components of, 36-37

Fourth heart sound,—cont'd
  differentiating
    from S_1, 73
    from split S_1, 37
  nomenclature of, 36
Frequency
  of heart sounds, determination of, 4-5
  of murmurs, 50
  of sound, 10
Friction rubs, 85-91
  pericardial, 86-87; *see also* Pericardial
    friction rubs
    and pleural, differentiating, 89
  pleural, 87-88

G

Gallop
  atrial, 36; *see also* Fourth heart sound
  presystolic, 36; *see also* Fourth heart
    sound
  protodiastolic, 42; *see also* Third heart
    sound
  summation, 43
  ventricular, 42; *see also* Third heart
    sound
Grip, hand, murmurs and, 52

H

Hand grip, murmurs and, 52
"Harsh" murmurs, 50
Harvey, William, 2
Heart block, third-degree, causing wide
    split S_1, 70
Heart failure, congestive
  fixed split S_2 in, 80
  S_3 and, 42, 43
Heart murmurs; *see* Murmurs
Heart sounds, 6
  and cardiac cycle, relationship
    between, 8
  charting, 12, 13
  classification of, 12
  first; *see* First heart sound
  fourth; *see* Fourth heart sound
  frequency of, determination of, 4-5
  left, 8
  mimicking, 15
  production of, 8-9
  recording, 13, 14
  right, 8

Heart sounds,—cont'd
  second; *see* Second heart sound
  third; *see* Third heart sound
  transmission of, 10-12
Heart
  auscultation of; *see* Auscultation
  damage to, and intensity of S_1, 22
  disease of, S_3 and, 42
  pressure curves of, 6
  primary disease of, and S_4, 36
  valves of; *see* Valves of heart
High-amplitude sound waves, 10
High frequency of sound, 10
High-frequency sounds, auscultation for,
  4
Hippocrates, 2
Holo murmur, 50
Holosystolic murmurs, 57-58
Hypertension
  pulmonary, pulmonic ejection sounds
    in, 70
  pulmonic, and S_4, 36-37
  severe, and S_4, 36
Hyperthyroidism
  innocent systolic murmurs in, 57
  pulmonic ejection sounds in, 70

I

Idiopathic dilation of pulmonary artery,
    wide split S_2 in, 79
Incompetent heart valve
  diastolic murmurs caused by, 64
  S_3 and, 42
  systolic murmur with, 56
Infarction, myocardial
  and intensity of S_1, 22
  causing pericardial friction rubs, 86
  and S_4, 36
Infections, viral, causing pleural friction
    rubs, 88
Infective pericarditis causing pericardial
    friction rubs, 86
Inhalation of amyl nitrate, murmurs and,
    52
Innocent systolic murmurs, 56
  causes of, 56, 57
Inspiration
  pericardial friction rubs in, 87
  pleural friction rubs in, 88

Insufficiency
   aortic, aortic ejection sounds in, 71
   of first heart sound, 21-23
   mitral
      systolic murmur with, 56
      wide split S_2 in, 79
   tricuspid, systolic murmur with, 56
Intensity
   of murmurs, 48-49
   of sound, 10
Intercostal spaces, as sites of auscultation,
   5
Interventricular septal defects, systolic
   murmur with, 56
Isovolumic contraction phase of
   ventricular systole, 7
Isovolumic relaxation phase of
   ventricular diastole, 7

L

Laennec, René, 2
Late diastolic murmurs, 65
Late filling phase of ventricular diastole,
   7
Late murmur, 50
Late systolic murmurs, 57
Lateral recumbent position, left, for
   auscultation, 3
Lateral sternal border, left, of heart,
   auscultation at, 5
"le" sound, 15
Left bundle branch block
   narrow split S_2 in, 80
   paradoxical split S_2 in, 78
Left heart sounds, 8
Left lateral recumbent position for
   auscultation, 3
Left lateral sternal border of heart,
   auscultation at, 5
Left ventricular diastolic volume,
   increased, S_3 and, 42
Left-to-right shunts, S_3 and, 42
Listening, selective, during auscultation,
   6
Low-amplitude sound waves, 10
Low frequency of sound, 10
Low-frequency sounds, auscultation for,
   4
Lower left sternal border of heart,
   auscultation at, 5

Lower left sternal border of heart,
   auscultation at,—cont'd
   "lub" sound, 15
   "lup" sound, 15
   "lupp" sound, 15

M

M_1, 20
   intensity of, 21
Mid murmur, 50
Mid-diastolic murmurs, 64
Mid-systolic clicks, 71-72
Mid-systolic murmurs, 57
Mitral insufficiency
   systolic murmur with, 56
   wide split S_2 in, 79
Mitral regurgitation
   differentiation of, by pitch and quality,
      51
   murmur of, 51
      maneuvers to differentiate, 52
   pansystolic murmur in, 58
   systolic murmurs in, 58
Mitral valve
   closure of, sound from, 20
   increased blood flow across, diastolic
      murmurs caused by, 64
   leaflets of, ballooning of, causing mid-
      systolic clicks, 71
   murmur at, locating, 48, 49
   prolapse of
      late systolic murmurs in, 57
      causing mid-systolic clicks, 71
      murmur of, 51
   stenosis of
      causing wide split S_1, 70
      diastolic murmurs caused by, 64, 65,
         66
      differentiation of, by pitch and
         quality, 49
      murmur of, 51
         maneuvers to differentiate, 52
      opening snap with, 80, 81
Mitral valve sounds, 8
Murmur(s)
   causes of, 48
   characteristics of, 48-52
   charting, 12, 13
   classification of, 12
   crescendo, 51

Murmur(s)—cont'd
  crescendo/decrescendo, 51
  decrescendo, 51
  decrescendo/crescendo, 51
  definition of, 48
  diastolic, 50, 63-68; *see also* Diastolic
      murmurs
  early, 50
  ejection, mid-systolic murmur as, 57
  frequency of, 49, 50
  general information on, 47-54
  holosystolic, 57-58
  intensity of, 48-49
  late, 50
  location of, 48
  loudness of, 48-49
  mid, 50
  pan or holo, 50
  pansystolic, 57-58
  pitch of, 49
  presystolic, 65
  pulmonary outflow tract, innocent, 56
  quality of, 50
  radiation of, 51
  shape of, 51
  special maneuvers to identify, 52
  systolic, 50, 55-61; *see also* Systolic
      murmurs
  timing of, 50
Muscle, papillary, disorders of, late
      systolic murmurs in, 57
Myocardial infarction
  and intensity of S_1, 22
  causing pericardial friction rubs, 86
  and S_4, 36
Myxedema causing pericardial friction
      rubs, 86
Myxomas, atrial, causing wide split S_1, 70

N

Narrow split S_2, 79, 80, 82
Neoplasms causing pericardial friction
      rubs, 86
Noninfective pericarditis causing
      pericardial friction rubs, 86
Normal systolic murmurs, 56

O

Obstruction, pulmonic valve, and S_4, 36

Open heart surgery causing pericardial
      friction rubs, 86
Opening snap, 80-81, 82
  differentiating S_3 from, 81, 82
  tricuspid, 81

P

P_1, intensity of, 21
P_2
  intensity of, 30, 31
  in paradoxical split S_2, 78
P-R interval and S_4, 37
"Pan" murmur, 50
Pan-diastolic murmurs, 65
Pansystolic murmurs, 57-58
Papillary muscle disorders, late systolic
      murmurs in, 57
Paradoxical split S_2, 78, 79, 82
Patent ductus arteriosus, 65
  narrow split S_2 in, 80
  opening snap with, 80
  paradoxical split S_2 in, 78
  S_3 and, 42
Pericardial friction rubs, 86-87
  auscultatory signs of, 86
  differentiating, from pleural friction
      rubs, 89
  etiologies of, 86
  sound characteristics of, 86-87
Pericarditis causing pericardial friction
      rubs, 86
Phonocardiography, 15
Physical examination, cardiovascular, 2
Physiological split S_2, 30-31
Pitch, 10
  of murmurs, 49
Pleural friction rubs, 87-88
  auscultatory signs of, 88
  differentiating, from pericardial friction
      rubs, 89
  etiologies of, 87-88
  sound characteristics of, 88
Pneumonia causing pleural friction rubs,
      88
Pregnancy, innocent systolic murmurs in,
      57
Premature beats, ventricular, causing
      wide split S_1, 70
Pressure curves of heart, 6

Presystolic gallop, 36; *see also* Fourth heart sound
Presystolic murmur, 65
Primary heart disease and S$_4$, 36
Prolapse, mitral valve, causing mid-systolic clicks, 71
Protodiastolic gallop, 42; *see also* Third heart sound
Pulmonary artery
    enlargement of, pulmonic ejection sounds in, 70
    idiopathic dilation of, wide split S$_2$ in, 79
Pulmonary embolism
    causing pleural friction rubs, 88
    pulmonic ejection sounds in, 70
    wide split S$_2$ in, 79
Pulmonary hypertension, pulmonic ejection sounds in, 70
Pulmonary outflow tract, increased flow of, differentiation of, by pitch and quality, 51
Pulmonary outflow tract murmur, innocent, 56
Pulmonic area of heart, auscultation at, 5
Pulmonic ejection sounds, 70, 71, 73
Pulmonic hypertension and S$_4$, 36-37
Pulmonic regurgitation
    diastolic murmurs caused by, 64, 66
    differentiation of, by pitch and quality, 49
Pulmonic valve
    incompetence of, diastolic murmurs caused by, 64
    murmur at, locating, 48, 49
    obstruction of, and S$_4$, 36
    stenosis of
        mid-systolic murmur in, 57
        murmurs with, maneuvers to differentiate, 52
        pulmonic ejection sounds in, 70
        and S$_4$, 36
        systolic murmur with, 56, 58
        wide split S$_2$ in, 79
Pulmonic valve sounds, 8
Pulse, carotid, and timing of first heart sound, 25

Q

Quadruple rhythm, 43

Quality of sound, 10

R

Rapid filling phase of ventricular diastole, 7
Rapid ventricular ejection in ventricular systole, 7
Regurgitation
    aortic; *see* Aortic regurgitation
    backward, causing murmurs, 48
    mitral; *see* Mitral regurgitation
    pulmonic
        diastolic murmurs caused by, 64, 66
        differentiation of, by pitch and quality, 51
    tricuspid
        differentiation of, by pitch and quality, 51
        pansystolic murmur in, 58
        systolic murmurs in, 58
Relaxation phase, isovolumic, of ventricular diastole, 7
Respiration, murmurs and, 52
Rheumatic fever causing pericardial friction rubs, 86
Rhythm, quadruple, 43
Right bundle branch block
    causing wide split S$_1$, 70, 73
    wide split S$_2$ in, 79
Right heart sounds, 8
"Rough" murmurs, 50
Rubs, friction; *see* Friction rubs
"Rumble" murmurs, 50

S

S$_1$; *see* First heart sound
S$_2$; *see* Second heart sound
S$_3$; *see* Third heart sound
S$_3$ gallop, 42; *see also* Third heart sound
S$_4$; *see* Fourth heart sound
S$_4$ gallop, 36; *see also* Fourth heart sound
Second heart sound, 8, 29-34
    auscultatory variations in, 31
    components of, 30
    differentiating first heart sound from, 24-25
    intensity of, 31-32
    normal, 32
    physiological split, 30-31

Second heart sound,—cont'd
  sounds around, 77-84
    differentiation of, 82
  split
    fixed, 79, 80, 82
    narrow, 79, 80, 82
    paradoxical, 78, 79, 82
    wide, 78-79, 82
Selective listening during auscultation, 6
Septal defect(s)
  atrial
    differentiation of, by pitch and
      quality, 51
    opening snap with, 81
    pulmonic ejection sounds in, 70
    fixed split S_2 in, 80
    interventricular, systolic murmur with,
      56
  causing murmurs, 48
  ventricular
    differentiation of, by pitch and
      quality, 51
    murmurs with, maneuvers to
      differentiate, 52
    opening snap with, 80
    pansystolic murmur in, 58
    S_3 and, 42
    wide split S_2 in, 79
Shunt(s)
  atrioventricular, causing murmurs, 48
  left-to-right, S_3 and, 42
Sitting position for auscultation, 3
Skoda, Joseph, 2
Snap, opening, 80-81, 82
  differentiating S_3 from, 81, 82
  tricuspid, 81
Sounds
  amplitude of, 10
  characteristics of, 9-10
  classification of, 12
  diastolic, in pericardial friction rubs, 86
  duration of, 10
  ejection, 70-71, 73
    aortic, 71, 73
    pulmonic, 70, 71, 73
  around first heart sound, 69-75
    differentiation of, 73
  frequency of, 10
  heart; *see* Heart sounds
  intensity of, 10

Sounds—cont'd
  quality of, 10
  around second heart sound, 77-84
    differentiation of, 82
  systolic, in pericardial friction rubs, 86
  transmission of, 10-12
Split S_1, 20-21
  characteristics of, 37
  differentiating S_4 from, 37
  wide, 70
Split S_2
  fixed, 79, 80, 82
  narrow, 79, 80, 82
  paradoxical, 78, 79, 82
  physiological, 30-31
  wide, 78-79, 82
Stenosis
  aortic; *see* Aortic stenosis
  mitral; *see* Mitral stenosis
  pulmonic; *see* Pulmonic stenosis
  tricuspid
    diastolic murmurs caused by, 64, 65,
      66
    murmurs with, maneuvers to
      differentiate, 52
Sternal border of heart, left lateral,
    auscultation at, 5
Stethoscope
  amplifying, 11
  for auscultation, 4-5
  quality of, and sound transmission, 11
Stroke volume, increased, and S_4, 36
Summation gallop, 43
Supine position for auscultation, 3
Surgery, open heart, causing pericardial
    friction rubs, 86
Syndrome, Dressler's, causing pericardial
    friction rubs, 86
Systole, 7
  atrial, 7
  ventricular, 7
Systolic murmurs, 50, 55-61
  definition of, 56
  early, 56-57
  holo-, 57-58
  innocent, 56
    causes of, 56, 57
  late, 57
  mechanism of production of, 56
  mid-, 57

Systolic murmurs,—cont'd
    normal, 56
    pan-, 57-58
Systolic sound in pericardial friction rubs,
        86

T

T_1, 20
    intensity of, 21
Tachycardia
    and intensity of S_1, 22
    ventricular, causing wide split S_1, 70
Third heart sound, 41-45
    auscultation of, 42
    components of, 42
    differentiating
        from opening snap, 81, 82
        from S_4, 42-43
    in lateral recumbent position, 3
    nomenclature of, 42
Third-degree heart block causing wide
        split S_1, 70
Thrill, 12
Thrust, 12
Thyrotoxicosis and S_4, 36
Tissue, type of, and sound transmission,
        10-11
Trauma causing pericardial friction rubs,
        86
Tricuspid insufficiency, systolic murmur
        with, 56
Tricuspid opening snap, 81
Tricuspid regurgitation
    differentiation of, by pitch and quality,
        49
    pansystolic murmur in, 58
    systolic murmurs in, 58
Tricuspid valve
    closure of, sound from, 20
    increased blood flow across, diastolic
        murmurs caused by, 64
    murmur at, locating, 48, 49
    stenosis of
        diastolic murmurs caused by, 64, 65,
            66
        murmurs with, maneuvers to
            differentiate, 52
Tricuspid valve sounds, 8

Tuberculosis causing pleural friction
        rubs, 88
Turbulent blood flow
    factors producing, 9
    heart sounds and, 8-9

U

Uremia causing pericardial friction rubs,
        86

V

Valsalva maneuver, murmurs and, 52
Valve(s) of heart
    aortic, incompetence of, diastolic
            murmurs caused by, 64
    incompetent
        S_3 and, 42
        systolic murmur with, 56
    leaking, causing murmurs, 48
    mitral; see Mitral valve
    murmur at, locating, 48, 49
    position of, and intensity of S_1, 22, 23
    pulmonic
        incompetence of, diastolic murmurs
            caused by, 64
        obstruction of, and S_4, 36
    sites of auscultation of, 8
    stiffness of, and intensity of S_1, 22
    structure of, pathological alteration of,
            and intensity of S_1, 22, 23
    tricuspid; see Tricuspid valve
Valvular aortic stenosis, aortic ejection
        sounds in, 71
Vascular disease, collagen, causing
        pericardial friction rubs, 86
Ventricular compliance, decreased, S_3
        and, 42
Ventricular contraction, and intensity of
        S_1, 22, 23
Ventricular diastole, 7
Ventricular diastolic volume, left,
        increased, S_3 and, 42
Ventricular ejection, rapid, in ventricular
        systole, 7
Ventricular gallop, 42; see also Third
        heart sound
Ventricular premature beats causing wide
        split S_1, 70

Ventricular septal defect
  differentiation of, by pitch and quality,
    49
  fixed split S_2 in, 80
  murmurs with, maneuvers to
    differentiate, 52
  opening snap with, 80
  pansystolic murmur in, 58
  S_3 and, 42
  wide split S_2 in, 79
Ventricular systole, 7
Ventricular tachycardia causing wide split
    S_1, 70

Ventricular volume and mid-systolic
    clicks, 71-72
Viral infections causing pleural friction
    rubs, 88
Volume
  diastolic, left ventricular, increased, S_3
    and, 42
  ventricular, and mid-systolic clicks, 71-
    72

W

Wide split S_1, 70
Wide split S_2, 78-79, 82